I0704437

How to Fast

An Introduction to the Science and Art of Fasting

Alexander Vladim

Copyright © 2022 by Alexander Vladim

All rights reserved. No part of this publication may be reproduced, distributed, or transmitted in any form or by any means, including photocopying, recording, or other electronic or mechanical methods, without the prior written permission of the publisher, except in the case of brief quotations embodied in critical reviews and certain other noncommercial uses permitted by copyright law.

By the same author:

Drying With Water: How I Overcame Alcohol Addiction With Fasting

A mailing list for new releases-

https://mailchi.mp/c4f6565242a6/alexandervladim

I can be contacted via twitter-

https://twitter.com/dirtyteaspoon

New book releases will be added here as well.

Index

What is Fasting?

If you have chosen this book, you probably already have some ideas about what fasting entails, and perhaps some experience too. Alan Goldhamer of True North fasting centre calls fasting, "doing nothing intelligently." By pausing the digestive process and resting we allow the body to recover. A fast is a choice that is arrived at personally; it can be tough because many of us have lost the habit of going without food, creating a build-up of toxicity in our bodies that is uncomfortable to process. But at the same time, it's biologically natural- we are built to fast. As Dr Mark Mattson, chief of the U.S. National Institute on Aging says, "The way we eat now is built around three large meals a day plus snacks, but we're geared genetically for going extended periods of time without food and functioning well. If our brains and bodies didn't function well we wouldn't have survived."

The origin of the word 'fast' is the Old English word, *faest,* meaning 'firm' or 'stable.' From this root came 'faesten,' meaning both *to abstain from eating,* and *fortress.* It's an apt dual-meaning- fasting is a fortress in which you can shoulder up your barriers against physical degeneration and unhealthy pursuits.

We have become used to eating at our convenience. As hunter gatherers, our food sources would have been less stable, following a pattern of feast and famine. Our bodies are naturally adapted to this, storing fat in times of plenty and then using it as fuel to get through leaner times. We are built to go hungry periodically- our body fat is the very expectation of times without food.

A wild bear cycles through phases of fasting and bulking up every year. After hibernation, she wakes and eats as much as possible, adding fat and muscle to her thin frame. Bears lose up to a third of their body weight through the winter, and regain around two pounds a day when they begin refeeding. Before the mechanisation of farming, our pattern would have been similar- feasting when food was plentiful, and slowing down our metabolism throughout the barren months.

Why fast?

The philosophy of fasting calls upon us to know ourselves, to master ourselves, and to discipline ourselves the better to free ourselves. To fast is to identify our dependencies, and free ourselves from them.
-Tariq Ramadan

Why stop eating? Eating is pleasure, it's social; for many of us, it's a highlight of our day. But stopping eating for a time can also be enjoyable, and carries many other benefits. Firstly, you appreciate your food more. "Hunger is the best sauce," wrote Miguel de Cervantes in *Don Quixote*- it sweetens the deal and leaves us satisfied with simplicity. By taking a break, we can consider the choices we make around food, and examine longstanding dysfunctional patterns in our eating.

Your body's cells are entire living entities with their own metabolism. They require a continual supply of oxygen and adequate nutrition. When our cells are deprived, we develop a sluggish metabolism; tiredness and poor functioning become our norm. If we adopt a sedentary lifestyle, with overeating and the resulting poor digestion and assimilation of food; lack of fresh air, and adequate exercise and rest, our cells begin to degenerate.

As the natural process of cell replacement and repair slows, your body ages, its resistance to disease diminishes, and you become unwell. We may visit the doctor's surgery, where we are prescribed pills, but these have side-effects. Sometimes they do not cure, only mask the symptoms, or shift the problem to another part of the body.

We are eating unhealthily, and too often- and as a result, we are putting on weight, and getting sick. We're not necessarily encouraged to draw a connection between these things. The links are easily seen in the science- and if there was more awareness, maybe people would take it more seriously. Overeating is bad for you, eating too often is bad for you, eating the wrong stuff accumulates foreign chemicals, and never resting from eating depletes us. If we value our health, it is necessary to reverse these trends that have a detrimental effect on our physique, functioning and emotional state.

We may be adding poisons to our diet, toxins whose effects we enjoy. These take their toll. A toxin is anything that is poisonous to the body that has been stored because the body is unable to eliminate it at that time. The liver cannot process all of its daily load, and toxic wastes are stored in the fat and other places. An example might be a buildup of lactic acid crystals in the joints, causing arthritis.

These are the poisons that we willingly put into ourselves, but we also suffer from pollutants that we never planned to ingest. Our lives are lived in a kind of toxic sludge. Air pollution, contaminants in water and food, and domestic poisons are all abundant. In major cities like Mumbai, the air is a toxic soup, full of heavy metals that the body is unable to process. "We consume about a credit card's worth of plastic each week," says Laura Owen Sanderson. It comes from synthetic clothing, from our car tyres and other plastic waste. We swallow 3 lb of chemicals with our food every year, and up to 50,000 microplastic particles. French scientist Professor Barbara Demeneix says that we are living with so much pollution that, "there is no way we can have a normal brain today."

She believes the scale of the problem is vast. We are absorbing "pesticides, plastics, flame-retardants, surfactants [an ingredient in laundry detergents], things we use in the kitchen, in the bathroom- they're everywhere. We eat them, we drink, we breathe them in and we even put them on our skins."

"The mixtures to which we are all exposed have been associated not only with IQ loss (leading to learning disabilities), but also with neurocognitive and behavioural disabilities, including autism spectrum disorders, attention deficit and hyperactivity. These disorders are increasingly common with rising trends noted worldwide."

Our domestic environments contain volatile organic compounds such as formaldehyde, and there are traces of cocaine and birth-control chemicals in the water. Over the long term, the toxins we are exposed to cause damage to neurons, which affects connections in our brain. Pesticides have infected every level of the food chain, and have even been found in the body fat of Antarctic penguins. We take on these toxins daily- they are stored in the body and for our long-term health, they need to be expelled.

Our toxicity is proliferating like never before, and so it makes sense to maximise our avenues of detox. In fasting, one treats this toxic immersion. Instead of adding to the body- pills, drugs and toxins, one takes away, consuming only water, in order to flush away the poisons and allow our bodies to patch up the damage our modern lifestyle has caused. When you start to clear some of this backlog, and feel the benefits in your functioning, it incentivises you to continue the process.

There is a growing interest in water fasting for healing and weight loss. More people are turning towards this ancient discipline to treat problems that are left unresolved by other means.

$$\Diamond$$

A fast is an act of subtraction. You go without food and allow the structures of your everyday life to temporarily abate, leaving you with a skeleton of your usual life. Through these bare bones you can analyse the different facets. You see the furniture that you've placed around yourself for comfort, or out of habit. There is a clarity which guides us towards a better functioning. We can throw out the old furniture which now just gets in the way. To use carpentry as an analogy, fasting is a saw; you can't do *everything* with it, but you can't get everything done without it.

Some Benefits of Fasting

These are just a few of the benefits- it is by no means an exhaustive list.

Breaking habits

Fasting is a powerful way of breaking habits. Fasting helps overcome addiction; it lessens withdrawal symptoms and increases neurogenesis, allowing new behaviour patterns to be formed.

Food is one area where many people struggle with compulsions. Our eating patterns are deeply ingrained, and in fasting we can begin to drill down into the foundations. What does the body need, and when? As we develop our self-control through fasting, we are naturally drawn to foods that are healthier.

Brain Health

There is improved brain health through neuronal autophagy; damaged cells in the brain are consumed. This is protective against neurodegenerative diseases like Alzheimers. Fasting increases neurogenesis, sloughing off old neural pathways and fostering the growth of new ones, allowing the formation of new patterns of behaviour.

Weight Loss

The sensation of hunger is created in the gut by the hormone ghrelin. It is a signal to the brain to eat. The gut has no idea how much body fat fuel we have available. It's a simple system, triggered at the times we usually take food.

The way we eat now has hijacked this mechanism. We are self-programmed to snack at all kinds of times, and the signal is given more regularly. It is similar to having the low-fuel light on your car coming on any time that the tank drops to half-full. The message- hunger- doesn't fit the facts; we have enough bodily food reserves to last us weeks. Triggers for eating outside of mealtimes include stress, boredom and availability of food. Snacking skyrocketed during the Covid lockdowns, and continues to rise, though at a slower pace.

Leptin governs satiety and lets you know when it is time to stop eating. If you overeat regularly, eventually your body will resist insulin due to overload; leptin resistance is the first stage of insulin resistance, leading to obesity and diabetes.

Our body's needs are simple, but our brains complicate the issue. If we can disengage from our mental, programmed need to eat, our body responds and adapts. When you reset the mechanism, the body falls into line, and it will alert you when you genuinely need nutrition. Intermittent fasting is proven to improve self-control.

There is, of course, nothing wrong with carrying some extra weight. We are often shamed by the fat we carry by a society that holds up thinness as the ideal. We learn to self-shame, possibly even becoming susceptible to dysmorphia. There's no intention here to add to the pressure that so many of us feel to measure up- or measure down- to this fantasy yardstick. Can we let go of this unrealistic blueprint that has been stamped within our collective psyches, one which serves only to diminish us?

However, if we can shed some of this excess weight, we function better. Duane Mellor, a researcher and teaching fellow at Aston University Medical School, says that losing just half a stone brings many immediate benefits. Metabolic and joint health improve; and resistance to disease is greatly improved with even relatively small weight loss. According to Roy Taylor, professor of medicine and metabolism at Newcastle University, the benefits of moderate weight loss include lower cholesterol, improved sleep, and a reduction in back pain.

Fasting increases norepinephrine- a chemical messenger that transmits nerve signals to other cells, such a muscle, nerve or gland cells. It increases the body's metabolism and increases the burning of fat for fuel. There is a decrease in adipose tissue- energy stored in the form of fat.

As well as reducing external fat, fasting attacks the fatty deposits that build up in the veins and contribute to heart disease. A study of more than 4,500 men and women found that those who fasted had a 39% lower risk of receiving a diagnosis of coronary artery disease.

Weight loss that has been initiated by fasting tends to be maintained. After a prolonged fast, there is a preference by the body for fats, which are not stored, but quickly oxidised. At the same time, glucose is less desired, with small amounts of sugar satisfying the body's needs. This results in less desire for food overall.

As one's regular appetite decreases after a fast, the body's food cues become more in tune with natural needs. There is improvement in the variety of the gut microbiome, aiding digestion and combating obesity. Overeating becomes less of an issue. If everyone on the planet were to live a western lifestyle, we would not have the resources to sustain it, but by simplifying needs and food choices, I believe fasting is part of the solution to environmental issues.

Insulin

Restricting the amount of calories consumed improves age-related insulin sensitivity. Insulin is a hormone produced in the pancreas that regulates the way sugar is processed for energy. In a 2017 UK study, diabetics were allocated to either a control group, receiving standard care, or a programme of calorie restriction to 800 calories per day. After a year, the diabetics who had adhered to the strictly limited diet no longer needed diabetic drugs to control their condition, showing the beneficial effect of caloric restriction on type 2 diabetes.

One study showed that pre-diabetics, when eating on a schedule between the hours of 7am and 3pm, and fasting for the rest of the time successfully lowered their insulin levels.

Mood

Mood is something that noticeably improves on a fast; fasting is proven to lessen depression in those who are susceptible. Herbert Shelton speaks of a doctor who had decided to end his life by starving himself, but found that as his fast continued, his mood got lighter until he no longer had any desire to die.

Ageing

Fasting reverses degeneration, by enlisting the natural healing force in us. It restores many of the impairments of age, changing the script that time has written on our bodies.

Linked to ageing, free radicals are inherently unstable and can damage cell function, contributing to disease. In alternate day fasting, cells produce more copies of a gene called SIRT3, which is part of a system that functions to inhibit the creation of free radicals and improves systems of cellular repair.

A study by Dr. Ming-Hui Zou, a professor at Georgia State University demonstrated that fasting causes the activation of a molecule that delays ageing of the veins. Prolonged fasting increases cellular resistance to toxins, if fasting for more than 48 hours. It activates pathways which improve resistance to toxins and stress at the cellular level, in both mice and humans.

Switching between fuel sources, (known as intermittent metabolic switching) such as when moving from glucose to ketones, followed by a rest period improves neuronal functioning throughout one's lifespan, with a particular effect on mood and cognition.

Fasting affects nad+, a strong anti-aging chemical. Nad+ repairs damage to DNA allows cells to create energy, protecting them from oxidative stress.

On a fast, small wrinkles on the face are smoothed out, and skin is rejuvenated. Bones and teeth become stronger. Scars can fade, soften or go completely, and anecdotally, moles are said to have disappeared.

There are fewer side effects from chemotherapy, indicating a stronger immune system that is better able to cope with physiological stressors.

The internal organs are cleansed. The digestive system, which rarely gets a break, can thoroughly flush itself, and therefore digestion is much improved after a prolonged fast. Internal scarring is also aided by fasting. As long as the organ is not atrophied beyond repair, then internal scars can be healed, according to surgeons.

Fasting is the most advanced healing strategy-its simplicity belies its effectiveness. According to Valter Longo, fasting for three days could regenerate the entire immune system. This has major implications for the elderly, whose immune systems may be weaker. Fasting triggers stem cell regeneration of a damaged immune system, killing older and damaged immune cells and generating fresh ones. The biggest causes of stress for Americans have been listed by a major study from Stanford Graduate School of Business and include a lack of health insurance at number one as the largest overall cause. Fasting is health insurance, a go-to for recovery that improves a myriad of conditions. In a 2014 study by Walter Longo, fasting triggered the creation of new white blood cells, a key component of the immune system. In various studies, fasting has been demonstrated to have a positive effect on hypertension, and strengthening the heart.

Eyesight improves- I have read accounts from people who wore glasses, waking up one day of the fast and simply not needing them any more, and there are studies which support this.

Robin Mesnage, a researcher into the human gut microbiome, has found that fasting browns white adipose tissue- unhealthy white adipose tissue takes on the attributes of brown adipose- a healthy fat- and begins to clean up the other white adipose.

Fasting improves arthritis, cancer and asthma. Arthritis pain is greatly reduced- I know this from my own experience. Fasting dissolves the crystals and afterwards the joints feel hugely better. Fasting pours new strength into the old frame, as caloric restriction slows the ageing process. Calorie restriction also increases life span. Monkeys who have eaten less than half of their usual food intake will live for up to thirty per cent longer, look more youthful and have more energy than monkeys of the same age who have not eaten a restricted diet.

There is no cut-off point for fasting- it still has benefits in later life. A study of adults over sixty found that intermittent fasting improved the functioning of their memory as their insulin levels decreased.

Fasting can heal things that many believe are incurable. "High blood pressure cannot be cured," claims the website of the American Heart Association. "But it can be managed." In fact, blood pressure is one of the conditions that can be normalised surprisingly quickly on a fast. If it is too low then it will tend to rise; too high and it steadily drops through the fast; in both cases reaching a balance in the normal range. The proof is in your own experience; when an ailment that has been paining you for years clears up, the joy doesn't need proof.

Money and the Fast

An unusual one, this- fasting saves you money. If you fast fourteen days, the cash you would have spent on food builds up in your account instead. You're swapping body fat for money. After a 26 day fast, I found I had saved enough to have a short holiday. It's not a reason to do it, but it is a bonus.

The betting firm William Hill used to take bets on dramatic weight loss. In 2011 a young man from Lancashire went from 21st to 14st and was paid out £10,000. He had staked £100 at odds of 100/1. Sadly, the bookmakers have largely abandoned these types of bets, having lost out too many times to keen dieters. I myself lost around six stone in a twelve month period in 2013, before I knew such a bet was possible. I didn't mind. My reward was health; discovering the power of fasting for myself, a priceless gift.

Mental Clarity

Mental clarity sharpens throughout the fast. Often there can be insights into one's life- new directions to explore or solutions to problems. In one study, fasting was found to improve alertness, emotional state and self-reported feelings of contentment, with a rise too in cognitive performance. A 2016 study of amateur weightlifters, found that fasting improved mental flexibility and set-shifting- the ability to shift attention between different tasks.

Buddha speaks of diamond mind, that like a diamond-cutting blade, can pierce all confusions. The diamond mind is free of obstructions, a state of pure clarity. Fasting brings one to this state- the mind is unclear at first, as old substances enter the bloodstream, but soon it clears like a gold-hunter's pan, showing the treasure hidden beneath. As Lao Tzu says in the Tao te Ching, "Who is there that can make muddy water clear? But if allowed to remain still, it will gradually become clear of itself."

Fasting has been used to help heal psychiatric conditions; in a study with schizophrenics, many were able to be weaned from their medication and rejoined society.

It sounds like magic, but there is a kind of divine magic to fasting; an indefinable, qualitative transformation. A mystic might refer to it as spirit; a revitalising energy guides the body.

◇

All types of fasting have an anti-aging effect. In a study performed at the University of Torino, scientists demonstrated how alternate day fasting increases the lifespan of rats; improving the protection and functioning of their nerve cells.

Switching between fuel sources, such as when shifting the body's fuel from glucose to ketones, followed by a rest period (sleeping, eating and resting) is beneficial- it improves neuronal functioning throughout lifespan with a particular effect on mood and cognition.

When animals in the wild are sick or injured, they will intuitively fast, and similarly, when we are unwell or emotionally distressed, our hunger decreases. This is a sign from the body that it wants to withdraw from eating temporarily, in order to focus its energies.

Fasting sets the scene for healing change and renewal. for me, entering the fast as a drinker, smoker and occasional user of drugs, with a poor diet and physical weakness, and exiting as someone who was free of alcohol, a non-smoker, with a much improved diet, a yen for exercise, and a newly-positive mindset was astonishing. It still is.

If you prune a rosebush, it grows back stronger and with vigour. If you remove the negative and unhealthy from your life, that which is left is revitalised. When we get out of our own way and let nature take its course, we can heal from almost any situation. If a condition can be healed, fasting, given its head, will heal it.

◇

Fasting is a powerful tool, and the dangers are minimal if it is approached with the right mindset. Like rock climbing, it is not perilous if one observes the protocols and adheres to the safety regime beforehand. You can fast intelligently, keeping the guidelines in mind.

I love that fasting is egalitarian. There is no need for equipment, special tools or a prescribed area. Plenty of detailed information is easily available, as well as fasting centres and experts who can guide a novice through the process. There is no hierarchy of fasters, only people on the same journey with knowledge that can help.

Hormesis

The physiological stress endured by the body during a fast is essential to healing. Known as hormesis, it is the beneficial effect of something that would be damaging in larger quantities. An example would be exposure to sunshine. This creates mild damage to the skin, but produces vitamin D, a necessary hormone. Moderated exposure to strong sunlight is of hormetic benefit to the body, and so is abstention from food. Fasting is a hardship that is good for us.

The Stages of Fasting

If we break down fasting into stages we are better able to understand what is happening in the body. There are different adaptations, like changes of gear while driving. Many guides to fasting speak in terms of hours and days, but I like Isobel A. Moser's way of describing them in terms of physical changes, and have used an adapted version of her stages, as described in the book *How to Be Your Own Doctor*.

Pre-fasting

Pre-fasting is a kind of 'stage zero' of the fast. It's optional, but if you are able to, it will make a longer fast easier and more comfortable if you prepare it for two to four weeks prior. One eases out of bad habits, meaning that the initial detox is less of a trial. Some recommend cutting down or removing meat, fish, dairy products, caffeinated drinks, alcohol, prescription drugs, and cigarettes from the diet in the pre-fasting period; but for most people, eliminating all of these substances is hard. For someone with addiction issues, it can be that much harder, however any steps in this direction will reduce the over-acidity of the body, and lessen the effects of any healing crisis, making things easier when the fast begins.

I've rarely managed to do this- fasting has often been thrust on me as a necessity; the body commanded and I had to follow. Sometimes you choose the fast; other times the fast chooses you.

Stage 1. The Disappearance of Hunger

The first symptom on a fast, unsurprisingly, is hunger. When the first meal is missed, our hunger builds. It can be persistent at first; the hunger comes and goes in waves, peaking on the second day, and finally leaving on the third or fourth. We get to experience that feeling up close, right in the stomach.

Hunger is a taboo. There is great fear around going too long without food- for some this might be a meal, for others a day, but for most people the thought of three days without food is unthinkable, and would, in their mind, bring them to the brink of death. It can be empowering to realise the falsity of this, but the first time, it can raise fear in us. Do we really know what we are doing?

For the first few hours, the faster experiences increasing tiredness. The body begins to run out of glycogen, which is stored in the liver and skeletal muscles. One needs to drink water and rest as much as possible. Feelings of weakness are common, and it can feel like a case of flu is beginning, depending on the level of toxicity. In fasting circles, the first few days of hunger, headaches and tiredness are known as 'the suck,' though I like to think of it as 'the price of admission'. It is a tough period, but one suffers the difficulties knowing that the reward will more than outweigh the discomfort.

You tend to get hungry around meal times- it's a conditioned response, so one technique when planning a longer fast is to cut down to one meal a day a week before starting fasting, and you only have to face the cravings around that meal time.

Within hours of the last meal, the body uses up its stores of glucose. This is stored in the liver, and also comes from fats in the digestive tract. When the supplies of glucose run out, the body begins to use the stores of glycogen, a glucose precursor. Within ten hours of the last meal, already fifty percent of the body's fuel is coming from fat.

The body enters the early fasting state, which will last until around eighteen hours from the last meal. Blood sugar and insulin levels start to decline during this phase, and the body begins converting glycogen into glucose for energy.

As this phase draws to a close, glycogen stores are depleted, forcing the body to look for another source of energy. This accelerates the breakdown of triglycerides, found in fat cells, into glycerol and fatty free acids, which are then used as a new source of energy.

The body's basal metabolic rate reduces, and the speed of metabolic activity drops to conserve energy. The heart slows and blood pressure is reduced. Glycogen is taken from the muscles as an energy source, causing a feeling of weakness. The first wave of cleansing is often the worst, with the body taking the opportunity to speedily purge the most dangerous toxins. It is a bit like a house-clearance; you shift the big stuff out of the way first to make space to work. Later on, more fine-tuning can be done.

The breath smells bad now, and symptoms such as headaches, fatigue, dizziness, glazing of the eyes, and body odour begin. These can be welcomed- they are a sign that internal cleansing is taking place. Sleep is often disturbed, and may last for a shorter period than usual.

One needs to take extra care at the start. One study suggests that not only is craving for food worse during the initial 3-day hunger stage of fasting, but cravings for non-food items can be increased by up to 25%.

Stage 2- Acidosis

Acidosis begins a few days after the last meal and lasts for roughly a week. During this phase, the body excretes acidic waste products quickly. Most people who begin a fast have an abnormally acidic blood level, and when you switch to fat as a fuel source, you emit even more acidic compounds into the blood. De-acidifying the body is a movement towards health; it reduces inflammation, the cause or cofactor in so many ailments.

The five main pathways of elimination are mucus membrane- nose, eyes and so on, the skin, breath, and the two obvious ones, the urinary tract and the colon. Water is a universal transport medium for these- in other words, water is the carrier that gets toxins out of the body through these gateways.

This stage is characterised by fatigue, impaired eyesight, and even disorientation. The breath continues to smell nasty, the tongue is coated with an unpleasant mucus, and the urine becomes concentrated and potent. To stay hydrated, two to three pints of water should be sipped throughout the day.

Mild acidosis is common in our diurnal pattern. After the last meal of the day is digested, the body works hard to detoxify from the previous day during sleep; and as a result, people frequently wake up in a state of acidosis- their tongues are covered, and they are afflicted with 'morning breath', where one's mouth feels like the inside of a trucker's glove. After eating breakfast, the detoxifying process comes to a halt, and acidosis ends.

As you progress and adapt to the fast, acidic blood chemistry is gradually adjusted, and by the end of the first seven days typically there is a lot more comfort, as you 'bed down' into the fasting process. Inflammation and irritation of the tissues is lessened.

This prepares tissues and organs for major repair. Depending on how badly the body is out of balance, normalisation could take another week or two. Blood chemistry approaches a perfect balance, and the faster experiences an increasing feeling of well-being, which is punctuated only by the occasional healing crises disturbing the peace.

Healing crises are periods of intense detoxification, and can take many forms. A powerful headache, nausea, or a period of diarrhoea are all common, and do not present a problem, though they can be scary for someone new to fasting. One might liken it to experiencing turbulence on a flight. It is ok to ease off, or resume eating if you feel overwhelmed. The general advice is to not break a fast during a healing crisis, but for someone who is unsure, when the fast is in its infancy, it may be the best course of action. The fast can be returned to later; it does not need to be achieved all in one go.

A faster who has been improving may be caught off-guard by the healing crisis. They suddenly suffer a group of severe symptoms and feel miserable, usually after a few days of elevated well-being. This is not a setback, nor is it anything to be worried about; it is a sign of progress.

Ketosis

Somewhere around day three one's body has entirely run out of energy sources from glucose and glycogen, and is unable to sustain itself by running off glucogenesis. It begins to use the body's stores of fat, converting fatty acids into ketone bodies to fuel itself, a process known as ketosis (one can buy ketosis strips to test for when this occurs, which is something I enjoyed when I first began fasting.) This is the protein-sparing phase, where muscle is protected, and it continues until all fat reserves have been exhausted. Ketosis begins as soon as twelve hours into the fast, but after three days it becomes the main source of energy.

Vital organs such as the heart are protected during a fast. They are ring-fenced and the body does not consume them for food. When blood ketones are elevated, fasting becomes easier.

"I delivered a lecture on this topic to an audience of medical doctors," says Rose Anne Kenny in *Age Proof*, "and one retired professor of obstetrics and gynaecology was very agitated about the concept of fasting. He challenged the data, arguing that it couldn't possibly be good to have ketones. He cautions that this was something he always tried to avoid in his patients, particularly sick diabetic patients. Of course he was partially correct. Ketones produced because of illness are an indication of how ill someone is and are different to the ketones we strive to produce with wilful fasting."

Ketone bodies are low-inflammatory, which promotes the production of a critical protein known as brain-derived neurotrophic factor (BDNF). BDNF has been called 'a miracle grow for the human brain'- a fertiliser protein that creates rapid growth. This production helps restore mental clarity by nourishing the brain with essential energy sources, and increases neuroplasticity.

BDNF preserves homeostasis, creating balance in the brain. Its production tends to slow as we age, but fasting halts this degeneration. It may be possible that ketones themselves are the main driver of the BDNF upregulation effect from fasting and exercise. BDNF has also been found to induce weight loss in lab rats by suppressing appetite.

Many who are interested in health have heard of ketosis through learning about the primal diet. Ketogenic or *keto* diets mimic the body's fasting response for sustained periods, and provide some of the benefits.

Fasting does not cause nutritional deficiencies. Certain vitamins, such as vitamin C, D, and E, as well as several other metabolic products, may be slightly depleted on a longer fast, but by halting processes of excretion, the body recycles its nutrients.

The amount of ghrelin in the system peaks at eighteen hours into the fast, and dramatically subsides after day three, and fasting becomes easier. Ghrelin is a multifaceted hormone, manufactured in small quantities in the stomach, which stimulates appetite and regulates the release of growth hormones, amongst other functions. This reduction of ghrelin allows a person to fast comfortably for a long period. A person with no experience of an extended fast imagines that a prolonged abstention from food remains difficult, and they wonder how it could be tolerated, but when ghrelin wanes, appetite also diminishes and disappears.

Autophagy

Between two and four days into the fast, the process of autophagy begins. This is the breakdown of old sub-cellular proteins into glucose, to be used as a food source. The term literally translates as 'self-eating,' and it was first discovered in the cells of mammals in the 1950s. All kinds of bodily wastes are broken down and used as fuel; cells shed their damaged or defective components. Autophagy aids in the removal of waste at a cellular level and promotes the apoptosis (elimination) of damaged cells, enhancing overall functioning. Bacteria, viruses and waste products in the blood are all swallowed up and used for food. This process continues for the entire length of the fast, with the various residues being thrown onto the metabolic bonfire as the body burns up its detritus.

Fasting also promotes neuronal autophagy, a process in which brain cells recycle waste material, and repair themselves. The brain strips away old neural pathways and creates new ones. The health of the nervous system depends on this process, whereby old cells are consumed and new growth occurs. Without autophagy regenerating the brain, it will atrophy, failing to function at the peak of its power and becoming subject to neurodegenerative disease.

Toxins are purged from the body, through the pores of the skin, in the breath, and the excretory systems.

Weight loss, which can be dramatic at first, slows down across the span of a long fast, as the body becomes more efficient at converting and using fat. Loss of body fat is more noticeable on the face. We are used to looking at our face, and small changes are more noticeable. The belly seems to go down more slowly simply because there's more of it.

Stage 3- Healing

The third stage of fasting, healing, might take days or weeks, depending on the extent of the injury to the body. If you fast regularly, it becomes part of an ongoing process, and you revisit old wounds for deeper healing.

After the blood chemistry has been stabilised, the person is usually in a deep state of relaxation, and a maximum amount of vital power can be directed toward tissue repair and regeneration.

Healing occurs quickly. To the faster it may feel as if nothing is happening, as now the healing crises have passed and the internal work takes place smoothly. Tumours are broken down, arthritic deposits disintegrate, scar tissue and wrinkles tend to dissipate and fade, and damaged organs regain lost function in this period, assuming they are not irrevocably damaged.

Generally speaking, symptoms lessen as the fast progresses. If one is toxic at the start, then there can be explosive purifications. Diarrhoea and vomiting are not uncommon, nor is acid reflux. One has created an acidic environment in the body through lifestyle habits, and in the process of rebalancing, many noxious substances need to be expelled. However, as the more violent purges fade, a sense of wellbeing develops.

Fasting gets easier the longer you continue. I once fasted for twenty-six days, and when I was breaking the fast I developed a throat infection, leaving me with no appetite. I added an extra two days onto the fast to recover, and these were far less taxing than day one and two. If you fast regularly, reducing your toxic load, it becomes easier each time, and you find you have more energy at your disposal.

Similarly, the first few fasts you undertake are likely to be the hardest, as one is dealing with a lifetime's build-up of toxins.

You may find you have more energy after the first four days or so fasting, which feels weird the first time you experience it. We are conditioned to think that our vitality comes from the food that we eat, and of course, it does. So how can you still have energy- maybe even *more* of it- when you are not eating? The fact is, we are literally carrying food around with us, on our bellies, our thighs and buttocks. The fat there is food, and after an adjustment period, the body efficiently converts it into fuel. Digestion uses up to thirty percent of the body's energy, so when it stops, it's possible to have more energy than you do when eating a sub-optimal diet. It has to be experienced to be believed, and it gives you respect for the incredible, complex functioning of the body.

Stage 4- Breaking the Fast and Refeeding

Refeeding is the act of kick-starting the digestive process again after days or weeks of inactivity, and is as important as the fast itself. It is a crucial transition. It is possible to become terribly unwell if this period is badly handled; and if you were already depleted of health when you began, a lack of self-discipline leading to out-of-control eating could have dire consequences. One risk is to try to go too fast due to impatience. A Moscow man died during the refeeding process after a forty day fast without medical supervision, developing severe bloating from trying to refeed too quickly, leading to heart failure. As a rule of thumb, returning to normal eating should take about the same amount of time as the fast.

I urge you to treat your body kindly and with respect. I often hear people talking during corporate [group] fasts who say, I want the biggest steak in the world, and I also want the biggest baked potato in the world when I break my fast. If you do that you will hurt your body. When you break a long fast, do so gradually.

-Mahesh Chavda

Raw juices should be your first meals, then small portions of watery raw fruits can be added after a few days, gradually working up to whole raw fruit. I do not own a juicer so I have always ended my fasts with small amounts of clementine, chewed thoroughly.

There is a case for not initiating the digestive process with pure juice, as it can tend to pass through the intestines too quickly, leaving nutrients undigested. The fibre in a clementine or watermelon helps get digestion started again; the bulky matter stimulates a process called peristalsis, whereby the food is moved through the digestive tract by a series of wave-like muscle contractions. However, juice has always worked for me, so I am happy to stick with it.

It is recommended to eat fresh fruit and vegetables for at least three days after a long fast, and avoid high-fat foods when you are refeeding. We are habit-based creatures, and the meals we make while refeeding set the tone for what we will end up eating long term, or at least until the next fast. If cooked foods and 'treat foods' are gradually introduced, they become less likely to become entrenched as part of a new addictive eating schedule.

If you've been fasting a long time, you should ease back into solid food gradually. A fast of a few days requires less of an adjustment and can be accomplished more quickly.

Diarrhoea and constipation are common when breaking the fast, sometimes both happening in the same day. It is clearance and purification, dumping all the junk out of you.

For those struggling with food addiction, the refeeding period is a time where temptation can be strong- especially the first meal. The body is craving nourishment and it is hard to resist the old, imagined comforts of junk food. It is imperative to avoid these temptations for a while. Avoid the snack food aisle. Make a shopping list and stick to it- it's easy to fall prey to 'decision fatigue,' where the quality of your choices is compromised due to tiredness and hunger.

Remember that just because you have started eating again, it doesn't mean you are up to speed. You may have started the engine, but you are not even in first gear. You can still become exhausted by simple tasks several days after the fast, as the body readjusts. A prolonged fast has been compared to undergoing major surgery; you need time to recover. Strength has to be rebuilt- muscles may be underused and weak- digestion needs time to reboot. This cannot be rushed. Do not head straight into town on a clothes-shopping excursion or go on a bobsleigh ride. It needs to be a gentle transition from fasting to the demands of everyday life.

Stage 5- Integration

This is the final, ongoing stage, where the gains of fasting are consolidated and new avenues of living are explored. It takes place in the body, spiritually and in life-goals. It can be pleasurable to find and explore new avenues that were never open to you before- whether that is in improved physical ability, personal interests that you felt unable to follow, or simply a new appreciation of the richness of life. Fasting unblocks all kinds of limits that you had accepted as permanent. Integrating your fasting insights into your life happens naturally, but may take work too. There may be a passion for sport, for healthy eating, or for spiritual and restful pursuits. You might wish to spend more time in nature, or discover a love for Tai Chi. If your health has been compromised there can be a desire to reverse this; if you have had bad mental habits, an interest in retraining the mind can arise.

After a period of adversity one does not return at first to the previous baseline of growth- there is an increase. Fasting creates a kind of self-imposed adversity, and the improvement afterwards can be so much greater. A three-day fast increases the production of human growth hormone by 300%, and a week-long fast boosts it by an incredible 1,250%, but there is also a concomitant growth in the entire psycho-physical organism- in terms of ideals, behaviour and adaptivity.

There is often a desire to weave the art of fasting into your life, whether by taking longer fasts once or twice a year, or frequent, shorter ones. It becomes a part of one's bodily hygiene. When one experiences the benefits, it is not difficult to fast, especially if the body has adapted and removed some of the more toxic residues from the system. There are times when it is a relief to stop eating, particularly during illness. The idea that we need to feed constantly to provide our bodies with nourishment is a misunderstanding, and this is one of the surprising things that is realised on a fast. We have plenty of nutrients and energy stored in our body fat.

Some behaviours integrate easily. It is the most exciting time; a fast can initiate new ideas to orient yourself by.

We may be spurred to improve our diet. After a fast, the supermarket shelves can be seen to hold a lot of crap. A glance at the ingredients of some foodstuffs fills you with horror- there are so many additives, and you don't know what they are, what they do, or even how to pronounce them. I have a very bad reaction to potassium sorbate (also sometimes listed as E202), a common preservative, leading to nausea for up to 24 hours. After committing to fasting, I started to question the value of things that entered my body. If I eat this ingredient, what is it actually doing to me?

It also increases a desire for physical activity. In a 2020 study on mice, carried out by researchers at Karume University in Japan, it was found that rising levels of the appetite hormone ghrelin could raise their levels of voluntary exercise. Ghrelin did not only increase appetite, it also drove the mice to choose to engage in exercise and physical movement. Due to this effect, intermittent fasting could assist overweight people in maintaining a more effective exercise programme, losing weight, and avoiding chronic conditions like diabetes and heart disease. But what it also points to is a natural movement- *towards* movement- in adherents of fasting.

After a few fasts, the body acclimatises with increasing ease, and possibly with little dip in energy levels. It's a good idea to start small with shorter fasts, and move towards longer fasts gradually. Some problems need attacking little by little. One notable entry in the Guinness Book of Records concerns Monsieur Mangetout, a French entertainer who once ate an entire Cessna light aircraft. That is not something that you do in only one lunchtime. You need to pace yourself with big projects, whether you are healing a painful long-term illness or eating a plane.

My Experience of Integration After the Fast

When I quit alcohol after a twenty six day water fast, there was a space left in my life, where previously there had been daily intoxication. This space felt like freedom- it was exciting and not a little scary. I found that I wanted to become healthy, so I began reading about different diets and moved towards veganism and raw foods. Having eliminated a lot of crap from my body, I seemed to do better eating lighter foods- a few apples digested much more easily than say, a bagel with salmon and mayo. I also found I wanted to be fit and enjoy the movements of my body. I'd found it hard to walk when I was drinking; I had nerve damage in my feet, suffered from gout and arthritis; I was often dizzy, and I shook. Sometimes I wasn't sure if I was in my body, it was as if I'd found a pile of other people's clothes and put them on; my limbs only partly felt like mine and at times would not move in the way I wanted. The fast began the process of reversing some of these afflictions, and I wanted to explore my body more and get back some of the functionality I had lost. In the morning I would get up and put on music and stretch and jump to it, a daily warm-up. It gave me a lift at the start of the day.

I would catch the train to Alderley Edge, a country park just outside Manchester, which features a great rocky outcrop that rises above the plains of Cheshire. My goal was to reach this clifftop swiftly, with a strong twenty-minute walk up a path that is patchily cobbled and winds through ancient woodland. I loved this walk, as well as knowing it was doing good for my poor battered body. The air smelled wonderful after so long shut in a stale room. The colours of the autumn leaves, crisps of bronze and gold, splashed across muddy pathways between majestic, ancient oaks. I drank it all in. It felt good to be in nature, to breathe with the trees and streams.

The Grocery Store

I love this analogy. I forget where I read it, so I am unable to give credit. If you do know, please contact me via twitter (@fiery_tomato).

Imagine you own a grocery store. It's looking a bit tired- the paint is peeling, some of the shelves need fixing and the lighting isn't great- so you decide to renovate it.

You can fix it up without closing the store. The customers might be mildly inconvenienced, but you can work round it. You don't lose any takings and all the work gets done in bits and pieces. At the end, the store looks and functions better with the shelves fixed and new lights put in, but it has not changed fundamentally. Bits of dirt have been missed, small inessential jobs overlooked.

This is the healing process without fasting. It's good enough most of the time, and can be achieved without losing any of the opening hours of the store, or in other words, having to navigate some of the inconveniences of fasting.

In the second approach, you close the store for a period. You employ all your storeworkers to deep-clean the place, every nook and crack. You hire professionals to come in and build new shelves, cupboards for the storeroom. A signwriter designs a brand new fascia. All the walls are repainted, holes filled, rubbish and dead stock removed. You replace the old refrigerator, add an orange-juicer and install stylish new lighting to highlight your wares.

When you reopen, it is like the store is reborn. Everything looks fresh and clean and new. It is not a superficial change- work has been done to the structure and design of the shop, and the cleaning has rooted out even the most hidden areas.

You have lost some time as a functioning shop, but when customers come back, they are impressed by the zest given to the store- sales go up and new customers are attracted by the bright store sign and window dressing. Soon word of mouth spreads and your takings double.

This is healing with fasting. It is more demanding in terms of time and effort, but the rewards are greater not only quantitatively but qualitatively- the benefits are greater, and there are more of them.

There is nothing wrong with the first option. It is quick and it gets results. However, if you want lasting, transformative change, the second option is your best choice.

Simplicity

There is no barrier to entry in fasting. All you need is water and a place to rest. If you're going to do it, you can really make no meal of it!

Patience can be a test. It cannot be rushed- fasting a week takes a week. This encourages us to adjust our pace of life. We are encouraged to trust in a pill as an instant cure-all for everything that ails us, but the deep healing of fasting takes time and commitment.

One thing that is obvious when you abstain from eating, is the amount of food there is everywhere. It's entertainment. Down every street in the city there is a kebab shop, a pizza place, an ice-cream parlour and a restaurant. Sometimes whole rows of food outlets beckon, with their lights, music and smells, enticing customers to spend an evening dining and drinking. Food is social and it is leisure, it has evolved beyond mere nourishment to become a social ritual of bonding and pleasure.

We are accustomed to the richest treats from every nation. You can eat and drink like kings and queens of old, delighting in every morsel, every cuisine, every dramatic technique. You can eat grilled swordfish for lunch, sushi for dinner, and, were you to desire it, a cockatrice for supper.

Fasting jams a stick in the spokes of this indulgence. There is nothing wrong with enjoying opulent treats, but when you are fasting, you crave the simplest meals, and this can feel like a relief. It is a palette cleanser, and a delightful respite from your appetite. It halts the cycle of ever-increasing desire. Is it not easier, instead of achieving your wishes to have ever more and greater things, to simply be happy with less? In addition, this is healthier as well. When we demand that complex processes are applied to our dishes, and a dazzling array of ingredients added, it affects our digestion for the worse. Being happy with modest foods is better for us.

On a fast, you notice how busy people are. You might be enjoying a conversation with someone and they abruptly dash off- they have other fish to fry. You literally have no fish to fry, and it is luxurious to have this space to rest. We are accustomed to so much activity packed into our days, and fasting provides a way of doing less and being comfortable with it, temporarily disengaging from the hamster wheel of constant busyness, with its struggles and stress.

Different Ways to Fast

People fast for many reasons- for health, for longevity, or simply order to lose weight. When undertaken for spiritual reasons, fasting can be defined as going without food in order to purify one's motivations and become more aligned with a higher power or God. People fast to find a solution to an intractable problem. Fasting can be political, as in the case of Gandhi or jailed hunger-strikers; or performative, such as David Blaine's updating of the act of the hunger artists, people whose remarkable thinness allowed them to make a living from being gawped at in a circus tent. Often people fast for several reasons- for weightloss and also to confront a difficult situation, or for spiritual purification and increased functioning. With the current popularity of fasting, many new approaches are being created and shaped.

Dry Fasting

The purest type of fasting is a dry fast, also known as complete fast, where no water or food is taken.

I must confess to some reservations. Dangers increase when one dry fasts. Its adherents are genuine and committed, but it's not something I recommend for more than twenty-four hours. We are already dehydrated. Most of us eat too many salty and water-lacking foods, and do not drink enough. Why would we want to dehydrate ourselves further?

The bulk of detox is done by the kidneys, and if they don't have enough water, the toxins they have to clear are more concentrated. Water dilutes toxins so they can be processed easily.

There are some dated Russian studies that support the healing properties of a dry fast, however it is the fast itself that is healing, rather than the lack of water. Water is a cleanser, it carries away the detritus, flushes the digestive system clear.

If we are dehydrated and acquire a pH balance below 7.4, we get overly acidic. This leads to anxiety, fatigue, and high blood pressure. Our blood is dehydrated and the heart has to work harder. Dry fasting is also more likely to cause urinary tract infections, as water is needed to flush bacteria away. There is a higher incidence of UTIs towards the end of Ramadan, as the protocol specifies that no water may be taken during the hours of daylight.

Water Fasting

Water-fasting as a healing tool has existed for thousands of years. Only water is consumed for the time of the fast. Many religious figures fasted at various times; Jesus went into the desert to fast for forty days to overcome temptation, Buddha fasted while searching for the gateway to enlightenment, and the Prophet Mohammed went without food often, including while writing the Quran, the Islamic holy book.

"Water fasting is the complete absence of all substances, except pure water, in an environment of complete rest," says Alan Goldhamer, head of the TrueNorth Health Centre in California. This resting from activity, including digestion frees up the body's energy to heal, and this it does; blood pressure, arthritis, kidney function, tumours, red blood cell count, sleep and stress are just some of the things improved by a water-only fast.

Juice Fasting

A juice fast can be a useful halfway house between eating and water fasting. One takes in juice-raw fruits or vegetables as nourishment. Typically, a juice fast will bring in less calories than a regular eating schedule, though there is no rule about this.

Juice fasting can be a useful halfway house between a full water fast and regular eating. You can drink juice mono meals, or blend up a selection of fruits and vegetables to give a balanced range of nutrients, meaning that the fast can be extended for long periods without too much loss of daily functioning. It is a less intense internal cleanse than a regular fast, meaning that it is less difficult to accomplish.

Mono Diet

A mono diet is a restrictive eating regime. The idea is that, by limiting what is eaten to one food type or even one specific fruit or vegetable, one creates more energy for the body to heal. U.G. Krishnamurti once claimed that he could get all of his nutritional needs met by eating nothing but tomatoes, which is exactly the sort of thing you'd expect him to say. ("Why is it?" asked my wife, unfamiliar with U.G.'s work- in short, he was fond of outlandish boasts, perhaps to curate his own amusement.)

A mono diet includes the grape juice diet, the potato diet, and the 'food island', where only one type of food is eaten for a period. It's healthy to spend a few days only consuming oranges- probably less so with pork sausages.

There's nothing wrong with a mono diet, but in my opinion it doesn't have any advantages over either a juice fast or a temporary adherence to a raw food diet, where more than one whole raw food is permitted.

Intermittent/ Alternate Day Fasting

Intermittent fasting is an umbrella term, covering many different styles of fasting, but in essence it simply means limiting how much, or how often you eat. There are protocols for fasting every other day, or two days a week taking in restricted amounts of calories. There is the restricted eating window- to restrict the amount of time in each day when food is taken. We might be accustomed to waking and getting some breakfast in straight away, and then not stopping until our last snack at suppertime. With a restricted eating window, we constrict the time available to us to eat. A common program is 16/8- you fast for 16 hours, and have a period of eight hours in which to eat. The most extreme version of this is OMAD, one meal A Day. Typically the eating window is one hour, leaving enough time to consume one meal. The rest of the time, the body is fasted. I've always found restricted eating window easier to stick to than other styles of IF.

ADF is alternate day fasting. We are into the more well-known and popular styles of fasting. One eats their usual meals one day, and the next a restricted amount of calories; typically 500 and 600 for a for a woman and a man, respectively.

Restricted Eating Window and OMAD

Another form of intermittent fasting is to restrict your eating window. You might see this written as 16/8 or 19/5- the first number is the hours in the day when you do not take any nourishment and the second is the 'eating window', when meals are consumed. A more restricted version of this is 'one meal a day' or OMAD, where the eating window is typically confined to an hour or so; enough to consume one meal. Some combine this with restricting the number of calories they eat, and add in a strict vegan protocol, for health reasons or weight loss. A restrictive pattern of eating improves the functioning of the physical system. The British entertainer Des O'Connor credited his youthful looks and vigour on his eating just one large meal a day, a regime that his showbiz friends dubbed *The Des Diet.*

We get a spike in blood sugar when we eat; if we eat three meals a day, we experience three spikes in blood sugar, which gradually return to a baseline over the hours following the meal. If we consume all of our food within an eating window, glucose levels are elevated for several hours after food consumption but then remain low for the subsequent 18 hours until food is consumed the next day. Ketone levels rise during the last 6 to 8 hours of fasting.

Intermittent fasting can be a gentle introduction. If you increase the time before you eat each day by an hour every few days, you gradually close the eating window, whilst minimising discomfort. Fasting is nothing to be afraid of, and we learn this comfortably on shorter fasts and eating windows. Try smaller gaps, you can get used to a small regular break in eating. You don't have to be overwhelmed with a huge undertaking. IF provides most of the benefits of a longer fast, over a manageable period that does not intrude too much on everyday life. One can potentially follow an IF schedule for the rest of one's life.

Sportfasting

Sportfasting is a modern use of fasting, aiming towards fitness and weight loss rather than healing. The schedule takes place over seven to ten days. You taper food consumption over the first three days. After this comes one to three days of juice, around calories a day, supplemented by additional vitamins. Finally, you enter the build-up section, where you slowly increase your food intake over four days, back to your usual consumption. Every day of the sportfasting regime, one does twenty to thirty minutes of intense cardio- running, rowing or cycling.

Combining exercise and fasting in this way improves body composition. It's also claimed that stamina is improved and recovery time is shortened, though there are no peer-reviewed studies at the time of writing- it's very much an idea in its infancy. It's exciting to see how this develops in the future- I believe that it will prove to be a very beneficial regime, as it mirrors the fast and famine plus exercise lifestyle of our past as hunter-gatherers on the Savannah.

'Dirty' Fasting

In dirty fasting, another recent creation, one takes water along with a small amount of nutrition each day. Some take this in the form of a bone broth; others start the day with black coffee, which has zero calories, or tea with a splash of almond milk. Others add MCT oil to the coffee, a short-chain fat that is easier to digest. Typically, a dirty fast will include less than 100 calories a day, blurring the lines between a fast and a very low calorie diet (VLCD) which will typically feature an energy intake of five-hundred calories or less.

Some dirty fasters drink snake juice, an electrolyte-laden beverage, intended to overcome hunger and keep the body's supply of essential minerals, such as sodium, calcium, and potassium, topped up. Studies of longer term fasting have not found electrolyte imbalances developing, but a small amount of salt can still be used to help suppress appetite.

Advocates believe that taking a small amount of nutrition, or zero calorie drinks decreases hunger and satisfies a desire to taste something food-like, making the process easier to accomplish.

A note about black coffee- caffeine is a mild diuretic, so this could affect hydration, but in the small amounts that are drunk it's unlikely to be a problem. There is some evidence that caffeine can also increase insulin resistance, but again, in small amounts this won't have a major effect.

A study into intermittent fasting casts a small shadow on the taking of additional supplements on a fast.

"One somewhat surprising finding," says Douglas Bennion, "is that when participants took daily oral supplements of Vitamin C and E, the benefits from fasting disappeared. It seems that because the cells were relatively sheltered from experiencing any oxidative stress that may have been caused by fasting every other day, they didn't respond by increasing their natural defences and improving their sensitivity to insulin and other stress signals.

This suggests that low levels of environmental stress from things like fasting are actually good for our bodies, and that antioxidant supplements, while potentially good at certain times, might actually prevent our normal healthy cellular responses in other situations."

Dopamine Fasting

We live in an age of distraction. Myriad screens compete for our attention; TV channels, YouTube subscriptions, texts on our smartphone, video games. Dopamine fasting stems the flow of information we are exposed to.

It is estimated that an adult in the 21st century sees and processes up to seventy-four gigabytes of information in one day; more than a highly-educated person in the middle ages absorbed in their entire lifetime. In 2011, Americans processed five times the amount of information every day as they did twenty-five years previously, equivalent to reading 175 newspapers cover to cover. We are suffering a tsunami of data. So much of this is white noise- opinions, adverts, irrelevant news, gossip and political skirmishes. This information overload is causing the average person to lose focus- their concentration is impaired, they have difficulty sleeping, and relationships, both personal and work-related, are negatively affected.

Severing the umbilical connection and fasting from information, from screens and news is one way to keep ourselves sane. Unplugging our computers and switching off our smartphones for a time reconnects us with the world around us. We may feel we are missing out at first, but this is more a symptom of detox than a reality.

To dopamine fast, pick an activity you want to target– emotional eating, gaming, gambling- and schedule a block of time to be without it, whether 15 minutes or an afternoon. If possible remove it from your vicinity- put the phone in a locked drawer, remove the fuse from the plug on your gaming machine, and so on. Fill the freed-up time with something enjoyable that is far-removed from the activity it is replacing.

In a sense, the term 'dopamine fasting' is a misnomer. A more accurate description might be 'fasting from habitual distraction or stimulation,' making a positive choice to go without.

"Retreating from life probably makes life more interesting when you come back to it…" says David Nutt, a professor of brain research at Imperial College London. "Monks have been doing it for thousands of years."

Fasting from News

In his article, *Avoid News- Towards a Healthy News Diet*, Rolf Dobelli suggests that news is to the mind what sugar is to the body. "The consumption of news is irrelevant to the forces that really matter in your life," he says. "News constantly triggers the limbic system. Panicky stories spur the release of cascades of glucocorticoid (cortisol). This deregulates your immune system and inhibits the release of growth hormones. In other words, your body finds itself in a state of chronic stress. High glucocorticoid levels cause impaired digestion, lack of growth (cell, hair, bone), nervousness and susceptibility to infections." He attacks news for breeding confirmation bias- what we believe, we will find reflected in the stories we read, which stymies critical thinking. He also believes that news ties up our minds with trivia, speculating on matters which are of no concern. As Nicholas Saunders puts it in *Alternative London*, if I need to know about it, I'll find out anyway.

Fasting from Speech

Fasting from speech often has a religious or spiritual intent. Vipassana retreats are held in silence for seven days, to allow for focus on the spiritual. In his autobiography, the actor Tom Baker talks of spending his teenage years in a monastery where speaking and even eye-contact was disallowed. After six winters spent in this highly restricted way it became a depressing affair and he left, craving physical contact. "My muscles used to crack to put my arms around something," he said. "A wardrobe would have done."

Idle chatter can be something that is refrained from, this being one of the tenets of right action suggested by the Buddha, along with lying, and divisive and abusive speech.

The Fasting Cure

A fasting cure is a fast of some duration, undertaken with the aim of healing a specific condition or disease- a fast to heal a chronic alcoholic condition for example.

The longest recorded fast was an incredible three hundred and eighty-two days, achieved by a Scottish man, Angus Barbieri, from 1965-1966. Barbieri was morbidly obese and was tired of the difficulties and poor health it created. His original plan to fast for forty days was extended as he found fasting easy and the idea of eating no longer appealed. He underwent tests by a physician every day, and took vitamins along with tea, coffee and water. At the end of his fast he weighed one hundred and eighty pounds (eight-two kilograms), down from four hundred and fifty-six pounds (two hundred and seven kilograms), and maintained a low weight for the rest of his life.

Religious and Spiritual Fasts

Almost all religions have some kind of story or discipline of fasting built into their earliest incarnations. Hieroglyphic scripts from Mayan civilisation provide the first records of altered states of consciousness arising from fasting. The Jewish festival of Yom Kippur traditionally involves a time of fasting from food, sex and bathing in order to focus the mind on moral renewal and forgiveness. In a retreat called *Vipassana* which is Buddhist in origin, participants fast almost entirely from speaking for seven days with a daily regime of meditation and talks on Buddhist philosophy, with the aim of self-transformation. The Essene Gospel of Peace, one of the gnostic gospels, advocates both water fasting and OMAD. Christianity has lent, a time of abstention to bring one closer to God, as well as the famous story of Jesus in the desert. The prophet Muhammad fasted and meditated, both as part of his weekly routine and during Ramadan. When a disciple approached him, requesting a deed that would aid him in entering Paradise, Muhammad advised him, "Stick to fasting, as there is no equivalent to it."

Daniel is the most renowned faster in the Old Testament. One of his fasts is described in Daniel 10:2–3 "I ate no pleasant food, no meat or wine came into my mouth, nor did I at night to myself at all, till three whole weeks were fulfilled."

The Buddha, despite turning away from fasting as a path to enlightenment, nevertheless continued to eat sparsely.

"Once, the Buddha was out and about with a large Sangha of his disciples, whom he addressed, saying;

I, monks, do not eat a meal in the evening. Not eating a meal in the evening I, monks, am aware of good health and of being without illness and of buoyancy and strength and living in comfort. Come, do you too, monks, not eat a meal in the evening. Not eating a meal in the evening you too, monks, will be aware of good health and..... living in comfort."

This is a time-restricted eating regime. Many Buddhist monks and nuns eat only once or twice in a day, and never after noon.

Fasting forces our attention into the present, where we have no choice but to acknowledge our hunger, our pains, our desires. We may suffer, but we are also in touch with the everyday miracle of being- a simple, joyful awareness that is often overlaid and obscured with thoughts and busyness. This awareness, unadorned, gifts us a seeing of the ungraspable beauty inherent in life.

The Vision Quest

A vision quest is a traditional rite of passage for Native American and South American tribal peoples. The method of conducting a quest greatly varies across different tribes- in one form, an L-shaped hole is dug, and the tribal member inhabits this tunnel in near-complete darkness for three days and nights, without food or water. The hope is to experience a vision that will give new meaning to the person's life, often from a guardian spirit. It can form part of the transition to adulthood, or be undertaken in order to seek a solution at a juncture in life. It's also a component of Native American ceremonies such as the Sun Dance.

The Sioux medicine man, Black Elk, tells in his autobiography of a fearful time. A young person of the tribe is never separated from the tribe from birth- now they are on their own, in darkness and vulnerable. It is not known whether it is day or night. This provides fertile ground for the vision.

"When the storm of vision has passed," Black Elk says, "the world is greenier and happier; for wherever the truth of vision comes upon the world, it is like a rain. The world, you see, is happier after the terror of the storm."

A vision quest forces a person to confront their weakness. It is a unique and powerful way to seek an answer to issues in one's life.

Ramadan

Ramadan is a sacred month for Muslims, who practise fasting, meditation, and prayer, and through this self-restraint hope to build a closer relationship with Allah. It is commemorated as the month when the prophet Muhammad received the first revelations of the Quran, and it lasts for 30 days prior to the celebration of Eid. The fasting takes place from dawn until dusk and includes abstention from water. Technically, Ramadan is a sustained intermittent complete fast, with Muslims abstaining for the hours between dawn and dusk. In Northern climates, when Ramadan takes place in the summer, this can mean fasting without water for eighteen hours or more.

The dry fasting in Ramadan is of a short enough duration to not be a danger, and the extra hardship involved in not taking food or water is a test of one's devotion.

Short Versus Longer Fasts

Both long and short fasts have their uses. A short fast can quickly address problems. A fast of twenty-four hours resets the body, and can be a starting point for dropping bad eating habits. When you fast for more than five days, profound transformational changes can take place.

Deep fasting doesn't always involve suffering, it can be enjoyable. I have had times when I have fasted for two weeks and had more energy and mental clarity than when eating regular meals. It feels strange, running contrary to the received wisdom of society. Around 15 to 20% of the body's energy is used to digest food; with this energy freed up you have more for other tasks.

Forty Days

Little attracts as much concern as hearing that a person wants to, or indeed is already fasting for forty days. I don't believe a fast of this length is necessary, except in cases of extreme illness that require drastic action. A professional would be the first person to consult in such an instance.

The idea is biblical in origin, and it can be seen as a milestone for the deeply religious, following the path of Jesus in the desert. It is achievable for a healthy adult, but it is a lot of pressure to put on oneself. However, if someone's aim is to humble themselves before God, following in the path of the prophets and saints, it may be life-changing. My focus is on health, and a forty day fast is not necessary for most people to regain a healthy state.

In 2006 a woman died on day twenty-three of a forty day fast, undertaken for religious reasons. However, it seems that the underlying issue was overuse of religious fasting for many years, leaving her in an undernourished state. Her mother is quoted as saying: 'She had been a Christian for a long time. She fasted frequently and would do it when the Lord told her to. Then she would start eating again.'

Dr Asker Jeukendrup, a nutritionist working at the University of Birmingham, said it was improbable that twenty-three days without food would be fatal to a healthy person of an average weight, who would likely be able to stand forty days of water fasting without serious ill-effects. But he pointed out that if someone goes without food regularly for long periods, the body becomes vulnerable to illness and infection.

With an unsupervised fast of this length, the dangers increase. Refeeding must be undertaken with great care. Unless you are facing serious illness and have exhausted all possibilities, fasting doesn't need to be done in one go. It is safest to have supervision, assuming a reputable fasting centre will supervise a fast of this length; most advertise ten to twenty-one days- a quite reasonable amount.

◇

The Practicalities of Fasting

Safety

One needs to keep comfortable and safe while fasting. At True North fasting centre, clients are not allowed to have baths, due to the danger of slipping. This is a reasonable strategy on a longer fast- wash with a cloth, or have a bed bath. If full body bathing is necessary, then take it slowly; you will be weak or unsteady to some degree.

Impulsivity

Fasting increases impulsivity, and driving is not advisable for this reason. It becomes difficult to judge timing, leading to dangerous situations. As a fast progresses you lose muscle strength, which also affects driving, there is a general feeling of weakness. Your concentration is impaired at times, leading to brain fog. Best avoided if possible.

One time I jumped a queue in the supermarket. (I sometimes suffer from terrible impatience standing in line to queue. It's a failing of mine, and at times I leave the shop wondering where that tidal wave of frustration came from. It's one area where I need to remind myself of my own advice.) It seemed nobody wanted the next till, and before I knew it I was scanning my shopping through- straight from the back of the queue to the front. The guy in front of me was not happy. He stood there frowning hard, a very British form of disapproval. If I hadn't been fasting, I would have waited, or asked him before jumping in. I think time had slowed down relative to my usual perception. Fasting makes you more aware and this translates as a lengthening of the experience of each moment, like when you were a child- there is a sense of timelessness. It was an awkward situation. I didn't learn my lesson, because it happened again a few days later.

Fasting Kit

It's good to have a fasting kit for comfort and warmth. Your body temperature is lower on a fast, and it is possible to feel cold even on a sunny day. I get chills in my feet, so I wear diabetic socks which are warm but do not affect the blood supply. You might also want to wear a hat, depending on the climate in your part of the world. I live in a rural village in the North of England, and it's sometimes bitterly cold in the winter; the nineteenth century cottage I share with my wife has Arctic winds blowing through the cracks in the doorways in January. Occasionally I have been known to wear a lightweight jacket indoors while fasting, a soft, padded one.

Elasticated trousers and loose sporty gear are good. Dress for comfort, not style- clothes that would suit an exercise class. I wear long johns as they keep the heat in. If your extremities get cold, you might consider heated slippers to warm them. They have a pouch containing grains, and when heated in the microwave they hold the heat for a long time.

If you wear rings, after a fast of any length they will become loose and fall off. I always enjoy this; it's a marker of progress. I own a few placeholder rings that I bought cheaply, and wear them until my weight settles.

Generally, the less weight you carry, the worse symptoms of tiredness will be. When I weighed fifteen stone (210 pounds), I could still walk quickly while fasting and remain fairly active. By the time I got down to nine stone (126 pounds) after many fasts, I was weaker. You are vulnerable in this state, and extra care must be taken. At the end of a twenty-eight day fast I realised how it must feel to be eighty years old and frail. I had to get the bus to the supermarket to buy food, and it was scary walking to the front while it was moving, and having to grasp the handrail with weak hands.

If you are weak it may help to have a bedpan or bottle to allow you to urinate- something which has to be done fairly frequently on the first few days- without standing up or moving too far from the bed. If you look upon yourself as an invalid this will help you to prepare and get into the mindset of a long-term faster.

Take care standing up on longer fasts. Due to the drop in blood pressure, it takes more time for blood to reach your head. A sudden change in the elevation of your head height means that the heart will have to work harder to get the blood to circulate there, so you feel dizzy or faint from a lack of oxygen. On a fast, the heart is slower to respond to this need. If you are moving to a vertical position from a horizontal one, take around thirty seconds, and do it in stages. I tend to straighten my legs first, and then raise my upper body gradually. One person died after leaving a fasting centre prematurely- against the practitioner's advice- and unfortunately died after a fall. Just because you have resumed eating, it doesn't necessarily mean that you are back to full functioning again. Slow movement is the key, care and patience.

How to Beat Hunger

How do you get through the hunger cravings? Paul Bragg says simply, "grin and bear it." The Times of India newspaper suggests ignoring them. Either way, the cravings fade after a while, forty minutes at most. It's a trained response. Ghrelin causes hunger to peak at times when we usually eat, around thirty minutes before mealtimes. Some fasters commit to a One Meal a Day regime before the fast, so that appetite is stimulated at this time and isn't an issue otherwise; one only has to endure the pangs around that one meal period.

If you're struggling, set a timer for two hours. If, when it goes off, you're still hungry, set another timer; but you'll probably find that the desire to eat is long gone.

Take it gradually, and set your intention. The hunger comes in waves, and fades again. Like any craving it can be gently observed with urge surfing.

Urge surfing is to focus mindfully on an urge or craving as it rises and falls. Simply hold it in awareness, and allow yourself to experience the intensity, without the need to act on it. Soon, the urge peaks, and fades away.

Length of Fast

If you are suffering a lot of pain, it's a good idea to break the fast up into stages, or adopt an intermittent fasting strategy; you do not have to do it all in one attempt. I have sometimes had to end a fast due to a migraine that lasted for days. I could not continue, but I knew I would fast again. Each time I resumed, the pain was there, but less intensely. Fasting took care of it, but it had to be done in shorter stints.

If you are malnourished, you will need to build up bodily reserves; the body can only use what it has available.

Prolonged fasting has its own rewards. One enters a state of equilibrium, where one is adjusted to the fast, and healing takes place on a deep level. Most people do not fast for a sufficient time to reach this level, and never experience the miraculous transformative benefits of fasting.

When to End the Fast

Shelton recommends fasting until completion, continuing until the body's fat reserves and waste material have been consumed. At this point the tongue is clear and hunger returns. I would advise against this, unless you have professional supervision. A knowledgeable practitioner provides a built-in margin of safety.

Shelton's reasoning becomes understandable when you look at his patients. They came from a background of serious illnesses which could not be treated by conventional medicine- people with cancers, with little or no prognosis of survival. For these patients, abstaining for this amount of time may have been necessary as an extreme fasting cure, a last-ditch stand against death. For most, it is not needed. Not every mountain climb is a journey to the top of Everest. Often problems fall away without any effort by the person.

Who is Not Advised to Fast

Pregnant and breast-feeding mothers, children, and those under 16 years of age are advised against fasting. People with very low weight must exercise caution. Anorexia is a controversial subject in fasting communities, and the ideal would be to first consult a physician. "One of my primary rules for fasting," says Jason Fung, "is that if somebody is underweight or there is concern about malnutrition, then they should not fast. I don't recommend that anybody fast longer than 24 hours if they have a BMI less than 20."

In addition, users of various drugs- anyone with a serious alcohol or benzodiazepine habit- brand names include Xanax and Vicodin. Abrupt withdrawal from various drugs is dangerous and this is contraindicated with fasting.

Diabetics are generally not advised to fast, though they are able to effect a short eating window, and there is a study that credits intermittent fasting with reversing type two diabetes. In this instance, a consultation with a doctor or other recognised medical practitioner should be the first port of call.

Fasting Supplements

I am something of a purist, though not as much as I used to be. It works for me, but I don't have an issue with others approaching it differently. What works for you is what works for you. I don't think people should be shamed for wanting to fast in a pure way with just water, or for adding all kinds of additions. It's a broad church and there's room for everyone.

We do not need to replenish electrolytes on a fast up to twenty-one days, as long as we remain hydrated and do not drink too fast.

There is a debate about whether it is necessary to replace electrolytes on a fast. Many say yes, as salts are easily lost through sweat and urine. Others, such as Loren Lockman of Tanglewood Wellness Centre, disagree- in his opinion, as long as water is drunk slowly, there is no reason for electrolytes to get flushed on a fast of less than twenty-one days. To my knowledge, there are no fasting clinics which recommend supplementing electrolytes.

I didn't use electrolytes for the first ten years of my fasting, which included several fasts of over 26 days. Recently I tried them, and haven't noticed the difference, though it's unlikely that I would even if they were effective. They are certainly not harmful, and it is one of those situations where there needs to be more research so one can make an informed decision.

There are many people who strongly believe that it is necessary. I watched a video by one fellow who was knowledgeable about fasting, and he was really selling the idea of electrolyte supplementation and then at the end he went on to promote his own brand of electrolyte supplements. Fair enough, if you believe in them, it makes sense to offer a high quality selection, but I do wonder about the promotion of fasting supplements, of various kinds. One reason I like fasting is because you need nothing, just enough warmth and water.

If you do decide to take electrolytes, don't take the pill in one go. Add it to your water so you are absorbing it throughout the day.

On Water

Water is a messenger, a carrier. If one looks into moist wound healing, one finds this borne out. A wound that is sealed with a non-permeable, watertight covering will heal up to fifty percent faster than one that is exposed to air. The damp environment promotes healing, and allows the body to easily remove waste from the area.

Some people add lemon juice to their water. It is not necessary but it will not restart digestion or throw you out of ketosis, so if it helps then why not? I have been a purist at times; when I first became interested in fasting I would frown at any deviation from the strict rules laid down by Herbert Shelton and other natural hygienists, such as the instruction to move as little as possible, and engage in no enervating activities, such as a hot bath, or distractions, like a tv show. (Enervation is the waste of tissues; a more modern term might be *devitalisation*, or simply *weakness*.) With more experience however, I have become a lot more relaxed about the process. So, on a fast I have had a warm bath, drunk herbal tea and read a book. Rock n' roll. If they help me fast for longer, they're preferable to ending the fast sooner without distractions, due to boredom. Fasting expert Jason Fung allows coffee, both caffeinated and decaffeinated, on a fast.

Distilled Versus Tap Water

There are various arguments about this. It is best to drink bottled water, or spring water, but not essential. When I began fasting I bought a distiller, for the purest water. Some adherents of fasting believe that distilled water will leach minerals from the body; others disagree. I'd count myself in the second camp, but there doesn't seem to be any firm evidence either way. My reasoning is that the body is intelligent and wouldn't dump useful minerals for no reason. Both camps are knowledgeable about fasting, so it comes down to a personal decision.

The Importance of Being Idle

"There is a curse of busyness upon the land."

This was a comment made by another attendee at an Advaita talk I went to. I love it, because it sums up a certain mindset prevalent in the Western world, of valuing action over recuperation. Dynamic go-getting has been pushed forward as the superior mode of being, a paradigm that Susan Cain in her book *Quiet* calls the Extrovert Ideal. We are swept along with it, whether it suits our temperament or not.

Rest is necessary, but it is becoming a taboo. To paraphrase Robert Pirsig writing in *Lila*, we know it works, but there's no way of justifying that because the whole cultural set up we have to operate in says that doing nothing is the same as doing something wrong.

In a society that promotes the Extrovert Ideal, it doesn't matter what you do, just do *something,* and be seen to be doing it. Society values those who 'make an effort', who 'get the job done,'- workaholics love their workahol. But not everyone loves the overwork regime- in a survey of 31,000 Microsoft employees, 39 per cent of them said they were 'simply exhausted.' Job insecurity and the need for an income keep us pressing forward.

Keeping on your toes is a strategy to not feel life fully. "We can blame the world all we like for there being too much to do," says Tony Crabbe in *Addicted to Busy*, "but really we're choosing it ourselves." We keep ourselves occupied, running away from a fear of what we may meet in silence.

In the city it can be hard to find a space to relax- always go go go! Everyone has seen those speeded up streetscapes of New York City, the cars flooding over the junctions, explosions of people swarming the crossings, the red tail-lights pulsing down 8th Avenue like a racing heart. Godfrey Reggio's *Koyaaniquatsi* has some beautiful examples. It's hard not to feel engulfed. When I quit drinking I'd go into the city and just sit and watch the rush and madness. I realised I could sit there every day for ten years and never make a meaningful connection with anyone.

"You become so busy that you actually stop feeling," says writer Brene Brown; we hop from one activity to the next like a woodsman leaping logs. Busyness has become emblematic of our worth as a human- as long as your diary is full, you must truly matter. Tobias Jones in *Utopian Dreams* speaks of "a caste system according to time and speed."

Measuring our lives by these standards makes us crazy.

Fasting is a remedy, necessitating inactivity and cultivating rest so the body can work hard on revitalising and resolving health problems. Rather than stretching ourselves to become, we stretch out in the sun. It's heretical to suggest indulging in the opposite of hard work- to recommend that we need more rest; more sleep; more breaks in the bustle of life. So be a revolutionary and have a good lie down!

We habituate to so much activity that it is only when we abstain that we discover exactly what our lives are composed of, and like a pebble in our shoe that we have learned to ignore, there are often parts of our lives that we do not realise are creating discomfort. By taking apart our activities and examining them, we can eradicate various long-term causes of stress. Fasting gives us a window to view those aspects, and put them right.

Fasting inverts the idea of effort; the body works hardest when we are least active. Fasting is a balm for busyness, and a cure for the over-complex.

It does fundamental work on our acquired tendency to overproduce, overachieve and overwork.

$$\diamond$$

Some people seem able to fast while continuing to work- sometimes it is unavoidable in this modern world. It is preferable to rest to gain maximum benefit, but the kids still need to be fed. The world is not designed for restfulness, and we have to make the best of it.

$$\diamond$$

When we rest, the curative work takes place with vigour beneath the surface. Like the winter, fasting pauses movement for a period, before spring's rebirth. It may seem that the earth is sleeping, but it is in preparation. Our bodies follow the seasons, and like the trees they fade and sleep, only to burst forth again. Fasting is the rhythm of our receding and regrowth.

The body is sovereign in fasting, and resting initiates vital healing processes, just as when we are ill. Energy levels shut down, often appetite will diminish, and it becomes a struggle to perform even the simplest of tasks. The body is conserving energy for healing. The less energy one uses in activity, the more the healing process speeds up.

Radical changes in one's measure of success or failure, happiness or unhappiness and wholesale changes in one's established associations, are resisted by our inbuilt stabilisers, and we often find ourselves pitting our wills against them. The will is seldom of much effect against the power of 'habit'.

To make the adaptation required by an irreversible change, after every effort has failed to restore the status quo, one must often retire from combat, slip into neutral gear and re-orientate oneself to the new circumstances that life has dictated. This sometimes requires an illness or an accident that immobilises the victim long enough to rest and realign his forces to suit the new requirements.

-Jean Liedloff

One time on a fast I had a healing issue of a running nose. It went on for hours, and I was ploughing through tissues. I went to the shops to buy water, and within minutes the issue from my nose stopped. The body had to use its energy to get me to the bus stop, and so could no longer process toxins and clear my sinuses. Such a simple thing had stalled the detox. This particular symptom never returned- at least until the next fast.

Fasting dovetails nicely with the Slow Movement and minimalism. On a fast, one is forced to decelerate and 'examine the scenery'. As Johann Hari says in *Stolen Focus*, there's evidence that a broad range of important factors in our lives are speeding up, including speaking and reading, and this is having a detrimental effect on us. "The images flash by so fast that they have to be assaultive to be noticed," says Advaita speaker Wayne Liquorman.

"What happens is that the senses become overloaded and numb." If we slow and simplify our lives we are counteracting this trend of acceleration, honing our ability to discern what, in the endless cascade of information, is important.

Fasting often works on Taoist principles. The rest from stimulation creates new growth. Deep relaxation promotes healing of the body, so that afterwards there is a greater joy in movement. Consuming nothing creates satisfaction with less. A desire for indulgence fades and one finds pleasure in simplicity.

Willpower and the Fast

Kelly McGonigal defines willpower as, "the ability to do what you really want to do when part of you really doesn't want to do it." After the desire to eat fades on day three or four, the fast becomes self-sustaining, the desire to eat created more by a desire for stimulation than hunger. It may sound bizarre but I used to watch the British version of Masterchef while fasting, a show all about creating novel and delicious plates of food. It wasn't masochism, in fact it's hard to explain rationally unless one has experience of it themselves. The dishes took on the status of a fine painting, to be appreciated.

Willpower is most needed when breaking the fast- this is when you must be strict. You are finally eating again, and you are in the supermarket, buying food, with treats of all kinds on display. Wouldn't it be nice to have some biscuits, a packet of sausages, or some French Fries? This is when you must stick to the protocol- or suffer unpleasant consequences.

Fasting aids willpower and motivation. In one study the subjects were divided into two groups- one in a fasted state, and the members of the other eating regularly.

Both groups were placed in a waiting room, where they were told that the experiment would soon begin, and while they waited to help themselves to a cookie if they wished. The fasted group were able to resist for longer than the non-fasted group.

The two sets of subjects were then asked to place their hands into ice-water for as long as they could stand it- a standard experimental test for pain tolerance and willpower. The fasted group were able to withstand pain for longer than the non-fasted group.

"Starvation Mode"

A lot of gas is talked about this. Some people believe that if they miss one meal the body will "go into starvation mode," but unless you're seriously underweight the body has enough reserves to survive for a surprisingly long time- at least forty days. Starvation is a serious business. Bereft of fat, your body consumes its own organs for food. At this point you are dangerously ill. One does not simply go into starvation mode after missing one meal. A healthy adult with normal fat reserves will not begin starving after one day without eating, or after twenty days; perhaps not even forty. Fasting is not starvation.

Anorexia

When there is a pattern of anorexia or avoidance of food then one needs to proceed in caution, and should seek professional advice. An eating disorder of this type, which is a form of body dysmorphia, can be built into the structure of fasting. Shelton advises short fasts rather than fasting to completion in this instance.

There are those who say that fasting helps with bulimia, and indeed, there are no studies that contraindicate it. However, it can be an issue- the misuse of fasting as a way of maintaining extreme weight loss does happen.

A woman commenting on a Harvard article believes that the warnings regarding the use of intermittent fasting in eating disorders are overly cautious. She says-

The disclaimer cautioning that people with a Hx [medical history] *of eating disorder shouldn't attempt IF without medical supervision is ubiquitous. However I have never seen anyone cite any evidence as the foundation for this recommendation, nor even provide clinical anecdotes or a thorough clinical rationale.*

I believe this is a disservice to those, like me, with a history of eating disorders. It has made experimenting with IF unnecessarily stressful. In my experience, IF has been the most profoundly effective intervention I've experienced for my bulimia.

It has totally regulated my appetite and normalised my relationship with food. My obsessive thoughts have completely subsided, my black and white thinking around food has gone, and I no longer binge! This is amazing. For the first time in my adult life I feel I know what it is like to have a normal relationship with food. I eat when I eat; a range of healthy whole foods and occasional less healthy foods, in normal, manageable amounts. And when my meal is over, I stop! Normal for others, a seeming impossibility for me (and, I'm guessing, others with eating disorders)... I think IF has amazing potential as a therapy.

-Thea

It's important to be mindful of the pitfalls, but on balance, there is little evidence of harm when someone with eating disorders engages with fasting as a therapeutic tool- as opposed to simply undereating- and anecdotal accounts are positive.

"Anorexia is as much about disgust as about control," says writer Jeanette Winterson. "Take a day noticing how bombarded we are with food– not just what we actually eat, but the advertising, the supermarkets, the sweets at the petrol station, the wrappers and litter and overflowing bins. A young friend of mine who used to be anorexic told me she hated how her parents were always eating– and soon she hated how everybody was always eating. And then she hated herself if she ate.

"Interestingly, the therapeutic clinic that I attended – the Buchinger Wilhelmi Clinic in Überlingen, run by doctors– is good for anorexics. There is no food– though anorexics undergoing treatment there are, of course, fed. But the doctors told me that the relief experienced away from food is part of the healthy impulse back towards food."

Motivation to Fast

Your motivation is the lynchpin of your recovery- your goal keeps you moving forward. It helps you to power through the first three days of the fast when temptations to eat can be strong.

One strategy is to fast for a long period to accomplish dramatic change. Alternatively, one can fast for shorter periods repeatedly and adapt more gradually. I like to schedule a mixture of the two, according to what I wish to accomplish.

You may find it useful to question yourself. What is it that I wish to change, and what is it that has prevented me from making the change so far? Allow time for the answers to develop from a bodily sensing rather than solely from the mind.

Take the reins, and you don't need to rely on another person or higher power. Taking control of your own healing gives it solid foundations. You know your decision from top to bottom, the *why* of it. When your sponsor is ill or your partner is away, you are able to resist temptation with fortitude, and that gives you confidence. Having been through a bootcamp of fasting recovery, you know you have the tools to succeed. It is the end of any reliance on a 'white knuckle' strategy.

"Once a person has fasted long enough to be certain of what their own body can do to fix itself," says Isobel A Moser, "they acquire a degree of independence little known today. Many of those experienced with fasting no longer dread being without health insurance and feel far less need for a doctor or of having a regular checkup. They know with certainty that if something degenerates in their body, their own body can fix it by itself."

In *Zen and the Art of Motorcycle Maintenance*, Robert Pirsig says he won't let anyone work on his bike because they will inevitably mess it up. He talks of once having seen a mechanic hit a part of his beloved bike with a hammer. It's the final insult. He rushes his bike out of there, and resolves to learn how to maintain and repair it himself.

In the arena of health, do you know what is in a pill; do you trust whoever is telling you that it is safe? Historically, there have been errors- not due to malpractice, but inevitable human miscalculation. There are extreme examples, the surgical knife left inside the stitched-up wound, the wrong meds given. What about the smaller ones that you do not see? What about the errors that are built into the system?

I'm not making a case against medical treatment, I simply accept that humans and human systems are flawed. When I broke my shoulder I went to the hospital. Once I'd had treatment and a diagnosis, *then* I fasted. The nurses were fantastic, the physiotherapist was skilled, and the doctor who treated me was entirely untrustworthy. Due to his egoism, some of his actions endangered me. As an example, he gave me the wrong diagnosis as a joke, a joke presumably meant for himself alone to enjoy. I later found out the correct diagnosis quite by chance from the head nurse. There is always room for human error.

By contrast, the system of fasting is perfect, because you are getting out of the way and letting the body do the work it needs to. Your heart beats around 100,000 times every day for decades, pumping eight litres of blood around 60,000 miles of blood vessels. An astronomical task, achieved perfectly, slowing down in sleep and accelerating when we exercise. How does it work so well? It is bodily intelligence. Like wound healing, or the body building new muscle during sleep, it regenerates naturally.

Fasting is the most efficient process of natural regeneration, and therefore the best method to combat disease. It is entirely compatible with conventional treatment, and at times renders it unnecessary. There is no reason not to make a synthesis of both.

Near limitless choice is stifling us, paralysing us into indecision in the face of a surfeit of options. Fasting is the antidote. By teaching us to get by with little, surviving on our own stored energy and avoiding unnecessary movement, it nurtures simplicity in our wants.

Fasting Difficulties, Criticisms and Myths

I discovered that the very thought of not eating makes people anxious. Food is comfort. Food is safety.
-Jeanette Winterson

The first barrier to fasting, and it is a big one, is the acquired societal unease at going without food for any length of time. The fashion for various forms of intermittent fasting have done something to dispel the myth of starvation, but still fear persists of the long term fast. As Paul Bragg said, "Eating regularly has become such an ingrained part of people's lives that, if you take food away from them, they experience many mental, emotional and physical reactions. That is the strong reason why fasting is not very popular."

Food is primal, it has been there since we were born. We need food for our bodies, and our spirit. Going without forces us to face whatever fears we hold about survival, about our formative relationships, our bonds with others. We have sought nourishment from our first day, and thoughts about it have been a primary focus of every day since. Whatever emotional problems we have are entangled with our eating.

Eating is often a habit, running mostly on automatic. We wake, we wash, we eat breakfast, then get in the car. It's done on autopilot and so when you break a familiar habit, you become intensely aware of the change. The awareness creates a sense of unease.

$\Diamond$

Not eating isn't much fun, until you are accustomed to it, but sometimes it's hard to get started. This is normal, your body expects food. It's tough. "In general, we want to take the easy way out," says Sune Lehman, "but what makes us happy is doing the thing that's a little bit difficult." The hard work of getting there can be offset by the knowledge that one is healing. We all make non-optimal choices and go off track- it feels good to set it right.

Fabrizio Benedetti of the University of Turin Medical School exposed two groups of volunteers to pain by limiting blood flow to their arm as they clutched a hand exerciser, a standard task to invoke pain in subjects without causing lasting damage. One group of volunteers was given standard instructions for the test, which merely informed them that the task might be painful, while the other group was told that the experience of pain would be valuable, improving their muscle performance. Thus one group was informed that the task would be hurt, a negative framing, while the other group was given a positive frame, that the task would improve them.

The volunteers who were told that the task would have a beneficial effect were able to bear greater pain than those who were merely told of the suffering it would bring. Researchers were able to establish that these effects were caused by higher activation of natural endocannabinoids, neurotransmitters that help with managing pain. By changing the meaning of the pain, the brain was able to change how it processed the communication of hurt.

A positive frame for fasting keeps us on track. People who are committed to a fasting lifestyle have resolved to overcome difficulties for the greater end reward.

I took a fast of three days out in California; on the third day I walked 15 miles, off and on, and except that I was restless, I never felt better; and then in the evening I came home and read about the Messina earthquake, and how the relief ships arrived, and the wretched survivors crowded down to the water's edge and tore each other like wild beasts in their rage of hunger. The paper set forth, in horrified language, that some of them had been seventy-two hours without food. I, as I read, had also been seventy-two hours without food, and the difference was simply that they thought they were starving.

-*Upton Sinclair*

Fasting can be a time of suffering, but the pain is both beneficial and necessary. Be assured that problems adjust and resolve- this is something that may not be possible to see until the fast is ended, when the sense of suffering, if it is present during the fast, falls away.

"The capacity to tolerate minor discomfort is a superpower," says the writer Oliver Burkeman. "It's shocking to realise how readily we set aside even our greatest ambitions in life, merely to avoid easily tolerable levels of unpleasantness. You already know it won't kill you to endure the mild agitation of getting back to work on an important creative project; initiating a difficult conversation with a colleague; asking someone out; or checking your bank balance – but you can waste years in avoidance nonetheless. (This is how social media platforms flourish: by providing an instantly available, compelling place to go at the first hint of unease.)

"It's possible, instead, to make a game of gradually increasing your capacity for discomfort, like weight training at the gym. When you expect that an action will be accompanied by feelings of irritability, anxiety or boredom, it's usually possible to let that feeling arise and fade, while doing the action anyway. The rewards come so quickly, in terms of what you'll accomplish, that it soon becomes the more appealing way to live."

Fasting brings our fears to the fore. They may be unnamable, but they exert an energy in the body. There can be an autophagy of emotions,

Along with emotional detox, there can be a purging of *stuff*. Unnecessary clutter might be removed, as we streamline our living spaces, mirroring the increased function in the body and mind.

Depleted Energy

You may be arriving at fasting as a last resort, as I did, with your body in a compromised state. It can cause discomfort to fast from this position; a poor level of health becomes an additional burden.

If one is fasting without supervision while the body is run-down and sick, it is best to err on the side of caution. One would want to avoid creating too big a shock to the system. Often a healing crisis can look similar to a bodily problem that needs medical attention, and it needs an expert to diagnose the correct course of action.

Fasting is not for every patient. Not every patient has the adaptive capacities to go through the rigours of fasting. Some patients require careful replenishment prior to fasting. In other words, you do not want to take a patient who has depletion issues into fasting because their adaptive capacities to hold up to fasting are limited. So we might go through careful refeeding and replenishment prior to fasting for patients who have depletion issues.

The fact is, just putting people on a plant-based, whole-foods, sugar-oil-salt-free diet is sufficient to induce intense healing response. It is just not quite as vigorous or as efficient as water-only fasting.
~Alan Goldhamer

Some drugs, if used over a long period, can leave the user depleted of vital resources and energy. In this instance, fasting must be approached carefully and blended with replenishing the reserves of the body. A more gentle intermittent or juice fasting programme might be best until the body has recovered some of its vitality.

In a 2021 study, exposing mice to repeated short-term bursts of stress was found to reverse symptoms of depression. The mild stress created in the body during fasting could, in the same way, be curative of previous depressive symptoms. However, too much stress is detrimental to a fast. Ideally you want to be rested- it's not something that is easy to do when under pressure from worldly commitments.

The prospect of entering a long fast for the first time can be daunting. Even a day without food can start to tower over you with the weight of expectation. So take it gently. If you feel you can miss a meal, try it and see how it goes. Perhaps even that is too much at first, but perhaps you can delay eating for an extra hour, and see how it feels. Get used to the feelings in you- is there boredom? discomfort? Does your stomach complain, or instead, is there a feeling of relief at the break from eating? Can you put your feeling into a few words- uneasy, tired, relaxed or irritable? All these small steps add up to a greater feeling of comfort around hunger. When we realise that hunger is just a signal, not an alert or a warning that we have strayed into hostile territory, we can start to relax around the sensation. If we understand some of the science around fasting, and accept that it is normal, that our body is equipped to not only tolerate, but benefit from fasting, and that it is something that has been a regular part of many people's lives for millenia, then we feel safe, enclosed in a new experience that the body is fully equipped for, where deep healing can and does take place.

Boredom

Immediately after a fast, boredom is rare. You see the world anew, and in my experience, the length of fast corresponds with the strength of wonder at the world. Simple activities like walking take on a new pleasure- in part because the ability has been compromised during the fast, because the body has been spruced-up and the joints revitalised, and because the lack of stimulation on a fully-rested fast creates joy in experience. Afterwards there is a freshness to everything, in the same way the air is vibrant after a thunderstorm.

Herbert Shelton recommends complete austerity on the fast. Whilst it may be the ideal healing strategy, it is not the easiest. A state of enervation in the body makes healing more difficult. For Shelton, enervation is the boogieman. His list of things that cause enervation is long, and includes hot baths, spicy food, loud music and social interaction.

Avoiding all of these may strike one as a tall order. Shelton, a purist, speaks of an ideal situation. As a blueprint it is fine, but you may not be able to fulfil every criteria, with the sheer amount of distraction available- nor is it necessary to.

"The issue of how much activity is called for on a fast is controversial," says Isabel A. Moser. "Natural Hygienists in the Herbert Shelton tradition insist that all fasters absolutely must have complete bed rest, with no books, no TV, no visitors, no enemas, no exercise, no music, and of course no food, not even a cup of herb tea. In my many years of conducting people through fasts, I have yet to meet an individual that could mentally tolerate this degree of nothingness. It is too drastic a withdrawal from all the stimulation people are used to in the twentieth century. I still don't know how Shelton managed to make his patients do it, but my guess is that he must have been a very intimidating guy. Shelton was a bodybuilder of some renown in his day. I bet Shelton's patients kept a few books and magazines under their mattress and only took them out when he wasn't looking. If I had tried to enforce this type of sensory deprivation, I know my patients would have grabbed their clothes and run, vowing never to fast again."

If you can do it, lying motionless with eyes closed is the most restful way to fast; the visual cortex takes up a huge amount of energy. This permits the body to focus all of its resources on remedial work. For those used to Vipassana retreats, with their long hours of meditation and silence, it's a breeze. For the less disciplined, and I count myself among them, it's a challenge.

At the Buchinger Wilhelmi Clinic, patients go for gentle walks in the grounds, which feature trees and lawns. While fasting you lose the sensual joy of eating, and their philosophy is to replace it with tranquil pleasures.

"What if I subconsciously planned to have a moment of weakness?"

Don't be hard on yourself if you break your fast before you planned to. These things follow their own timetable. There are many temptations to eat, and if you followed a compulsion, treat yourself with kindness. You can fast again.

Criticism

A couple of family members were critical of my weight loss after quitting booze. I was a healthy weight after fasting, and I looked better than I had done for ten years.

Friends were complimentary, but my family couldn't see it. *Are you losing weight?* they would ask, more an accusation than a question. Well yes, I was obese and sick, did you not notice?

Feelings about food go to the heart of us, and stepping outside the expected norms of eating makes people feel threatened. Fasting is the ultimate challenge to our accepted ideas about food, it rejects the cultural assumption that food taken regularly is essential for strength and energy, or that the energy of food is needed for healing. It is no wonder people find it difficult to accept your intention. All our lives we have been inculcated with this view, with very little to provide an alternative viewpoint. Recently, things have started to change, but there is still prejudice about even intermittent fasting. If you say that you feel weak from going without food, people take it as evidence that you are damaging yourself. They have no frame of reference, other than the information that has been passed to them.

The Buddha advised to suffer the slings and arrows, and let them fall away like missiles bouncing off the hide of an elephant. "When you wake up in the morning, tell yourself: the people I deal with today will be meddling, ungrateful, arrogant, dishonest, jealous and surly," said the stoic Marcus Aurelius, always one to see the best in people. "But none of them can hurt me. No one can implicate me in ugliness. Nor can I feel angry at my relative, or hate him." We can tolerate disapproval, because fasting needs no defence- the results prove themselves. When you know the benefits, the mistaken ideas of others who have not walked this path trouble you less. The faster is guided by spirit. She is a warrior, she goes her own way. "It is better to conquer yourself," said the Buddha, "than to win a thousand battles."

Others worry when they see someone they care about in the later stages of a fast, and this is understandable. One can look gaunt after a long fast. For someone who doesn't understand or have experience of the fasting process, it is an unsettling sight. Shelton says that your family can be your worst enemy in these circumstances; not through any disloyalty, but from a lack of understanding. However, when family is onside, it is a huge boon.

I had a friend who believed that going without food for a couple of days meant death. He told me this when I hadn't eaten for twenty days or so, and was still functioning normally, if slowly. He couldn't conceive of it, he simply had no frame of reference. A poster on an internet site stated that anyone who claims to have fasted for more than a day is a liar or a fantasist- harsh words from someone who posts intelligently on other topics. It demonstrates how fasting is still surrounded by myths and fears.

People have difficulty believing that going without food for even a few days is possible. But you are not without food- you are eating from a larder that is stored on your body. A packed lunch. It's the fastest food there is- you don't need to lift a finger to consume it. No chewing required. Small wonder it is so efficient in providing energy.

This stored energy is there precisely to support us through these times. Would we have survived as a species without fasting? A failed harvest, several abandoned hunts in a row, or the death of the most skilled trapper might have threatened the survival of the whole tribe. Consuming stored fat reserves is a way of smoothing over these inevitable lean times when living in the natural world. The mechanism hasn't disappeared just because we now live in an age with factory farming and convenience foods. Our fat reserves- and those of other animals that experience lean times- are the very expectation of fasting.

I love to share my love of fasting with others on the path, but I don't try to convert people who don't already have an interest. It makes me sad when people suffer from illnesses that I feel they could heal by fasting, but I never interfere unless they seem like they might be receptive, which is rare. However, there is a love of talking about it, reading other's experiences. Fasting is a beautiful thing to do.

They See Me Fastin'- They be Hatin'

There are some vociferous anti-fasting comments online; I see them in articles about weight loss and diets.

Every January, the same old battle cry: this will be the year that I get thin. Last January, I did a week-long juice cleanse, and the year before that, I fasted for three days. It wasn't quite nil by mouth, but almost. At the time, I told myself the science interested me (the fervour with which fasting evangelists assure you that a few days without food can reset your microbiome or stave off cellular ageing is compelling enough to make you ignore the health warnings). Really, though, what I wanted was rapid weight loss, minimum one dress size.

I made it to 81 hours. Practically levitating with hunger, I ignored the advice to reintroduce food slowly (soups and juices before solids) by bingeing on a cheese sandwich, which I promptly threw up.

From this, one learns the absolute importance of breaking the fast correctly. Even after a relatively short period without eating, the body violently rejects solid, high-fat foods. The rules of refeeding- take it gradually, beginning with juices- have solid reasoning supporting them. Fasting is not dangerous, but it does need to be taken seriously.

There is a dig here against 'fasting evangelists.' I don't consider myself one- I'm a realist- but I accept that I'm more enthusiastic than most. How could I not be, with the healing it has given me? The fact is, fasting *can* stave off cellular ageing, but only if it becomes part of a lifestyle change with associated dietary improvements. To fast for three days and then express dismay when you get sick from refeeding badly is like someone taking up jogging, deciding to run a half-marathon on day four and being surprised when they feel nauseous after two miles. Fasting can be used for healthy weight loss, but it is not a three-day quick fix.

I understand the frustration of the writer, and I don't wish to shame them- but it is disappointing when people with little understanding of fasting have a bad experience due to a flawed approach, and then advise others on this basis. To return to a favourite analogy, if I decided to 'have a go' at mountaineering and ignore safety procedures, leading to an accident, I might be wise to blame my own lack of adherence to basic safety rules, rather than the sport itself.

Following the rules of fasting can be tough, but they make the journey easier. There is solid reasoning to back them. Stepping outside the boundaries can cause unnecessary suffering.

Is Fasting Safe?

I have to say that in 10,000 consecutive patients, everybody who has walked in for fasting has been able to walk out. We have no mortality associated with fasting to date, and as our safety data indicates, this is a safe and effective process when it is done according to protocol.

-Alan Goldhamer

When detoxing is severe, it can be difficult to decide whether to power through the symptoms or take a break to give yourself some breathing room. It can be risky to continue at times, and a good rule of thumb is to always err on the side of caution. This is why having a guide or fasting specialist on hand may help you discern between a painful detox healing crisis and a dangerous bodily response.

Why fast? (slight return)

There are many reasons to fast, and hopefully this book has blasted you through some of the pitfalls and given you useful tips on how to go about it.

I hope to inspire people to incorporate fasting into their healing strategies, whether that be from addiction, bodily pain, disease or emotional disquiet. Fasting is a powerful strategy to face and solve life challenges. The tips shared here are things that have helped me over the years. The stages of fasting have also proved useful to me, as a guide for what is happening in the body. Once the hunger fades on day three, it's like you've done the work of paddling out to meet the wave, and now you can surf it.

Any fast, conducted safely, is helpful, is a net plus. If you go gently, you can increase the amount of fasting you can do, to address issues of health and functioning. Juice fasting, intermittent fasting, water fasting- all have a positive effect.

A carefully managed fast is the most advantageous way of healing. I know of nothing better, and I have threaded its fibres through the fabric of my own life. Most days I have a restricted eating window of three hours, where I consume my nourishment. This has been the case for so many years now that it feels strange to me on those days when I eat lunch, or even more rarely, breakfast.

I also undertake a longer fast most years. This can have life-changing results. For me, the benefits are often emotional, as well as repairing damage to the body and improving my thinking.

Fasting is fertile ground, and when you step forward with courage, you enter realms of healing that you would not believe were possible. As your pains improve, as your life gets back on track, as your worries fade, and your confidence in your ability to face any health challenge strengthen, you find ways to make fasting a talisman in your own life, one which will serve you all your days.

References

<u>Chapter 1- What is Fasting?</u>

Before the mechanisation of farming- Preidt, R., 2016. *Are We Programmed to Overeat in Winter?*. [online] WebMD. Available at: <https://www.webmd.com/diet/news/20160109/are-we-programmed-to-overeat-in-winter>

"We consume about a credit card's worth of plastic each week,"- Hayes, N., 2022. *The Trespasser's Companion*. London: Bloomsbury Publishing Plc, p.51.

We swallow 3 lb of chemicals with our food every year- Gibbens, S., 2019. *The average person eats thousands of plastic particles every year, study finds*. [online] Environment. Available at: <https://www.nationalgeographic.com/environment/article/you-eat-thousands-of-bits-of-plastic-every-year>

We eat them, we drink, we breathe them in and we even put them on our skins"- 2022. *Chemicals in our everyday environment 'are* *poisoning our brains'*. [video] Available at: <https://www.france24.com/en/20171223-interview-barbara-demeneix-chemicals-toxic-cocktail-poisoning-brains-iq-autism-endocrines>

These disorders are increasingly common…- Demeneix, P., 2020. *Letter: Chemical pollution is another 'asteroid threat'*. [online] Ft.com. Available at: <https://www.ft.com/content/16c21f18-30b0-11ea-a329-0bcf87a328f2>

…there are traces of cocaine and birth-control chemicals in the water- Withnall, A., 2014. Cocaine use in Britain so high it has contaminated drinking water, report shows. *The Independent*, [online] Available at: <https://www.independent.co.uk/news/uk/home-news/cocaine-use-in-britain-so-high-it-has-contaminated-our-drinking-water-report-shows-9350477.html>

…have even been found in the body fat of Antarctic penguins- Zabarenko, D., 2008. Pesticide DDT shows up in Antarctic penguins. *Reuters*, [online] Available at:

<https://www.reuters.com/article/us-penguins-ddt-idUSN0933540320080510>

damaged cells in the brain are consumed- Alirezaei, M., *et al.*, 2010. Short-term fasting induces profound neuronal autophagy. *Autophagy*, 6(6), pp.702-710.

continues to rise, though at a slower pace- Bakaloudi, D., *et al*, 2021. The impact of COVID-19 lockdown on snacking habits, fast-food and alcohol consumption: A systematic review of the evidence. *Clinical Nutrition*.

build up in the veins and contribute to heart disease- Kroeger, C., 2013. Improvement in coronary heart disease risk factors during an intermittent fasting/calorie restriction regimen: Relationship to adipokine modulations. *The FASEB Journal*, 27(S1).

receiving a diagnosis of coronary artery disease- Laino, C., 2007. *Fasting May Cut Heart Risks*. [online] WebMD. Available at:

<https://www.webmd.com/heart-disease/news/20071106/fasting-may-cut-heart-risks>

in those who are susceptible- Zhang, Y., *et al*, 2015. The Effects of Calorie Restriction in Depression and Potential Mechanisms. *Current Neuropharmacology*, 13(4), pp.536-542.

…at the cellular level, in both mice and humans. Cheng, C.-W. (2016) "Prolonged fasting reduces IGF-1/PKA to promote hematopoietic-stem-cell-based regeneration and reverse immunosuppression," *Cell Stem Cell*, 18(2), pp. 291–292. Available at: https://doi.org/10.1016/j.stem.2016.01.018.

…better able to cope with physiological stressors- Riedinger, C., *et al*, 2020. Water-only fasting and its effect on chemotherapy administration in gynecologic malignancies. *Gynecologic Oncology*, 159, p.13.

…number one as the largest overall cause- Lynch, S., 2015. *Why Your Workplace Might Be Killing You.* [online] Stanford Graduate School of

Business. Available at:
<https://www.gsb.stanford.edu/insights/why-your-workplace-might-be-killing-you>

…hypertension, and strengthening the heart- Goldhamer, A., 2002. Medically supervised water-only fasting in the treatment of hypertension. *Journal of Manipulative and Physiological Therapeutics*, 25(2), pp.138-139.

…and there are studies which support this- Daily, S., 2022. *Intriguing connection between diet, eye health and lifespan uncovered.* [online] Science Daily. Available at:
<https://www.sciencedaily.com/releases/2022/06/220607120954.htm>

…can be normalised surprisingly quickly on a fast- Shi, H., 2021. Restructuring the Gut Microbiota by Intermittent Fasting Lowers Blood Pressure. *The FASEB Journal*, 35(S1).

…with a rise too in cognitive performance- Fond, G; MacGregor, A; Leboyer, M; Michalsen, A (2013). "Fasting in mood disorders: Neurobiology and effectiveness. A review of the literature". Psychiatry Research. 209 (3): 253–8. doi:10.1016/j.psychres.2012.12.018. PMID 23332541. S2CID 39700065.

...it will gradually become clear of itself- Lao-tse, 2000. *Tao Te Ching*. Kbh.: Aschehoug.

...weaned from their medication and rejoined society- Cott, A. (1970) *[PDF] controlled fasting treatment for schizophrenia: Semantic scholar*. Available at: https://www.semanticscholar.org/paper/Controlled-Fasting-Treatment-for-Schizophrenia-Cott/542b4954547b280b2a12dcc3d0fa4525952cbda4

...improving the protection and functioning of their nerve cells- Castello, L., et al, 2010. Alternate-day fasting protects the rat heart against age-induced inflammation and fibrosis by inhibiting oxidative damage and NF-kB activation. *Free Radical Biology and Medicine*, 48(1), pp.47-54.

…a particular effect on mood and cognition- Mattson, M., Moehl, K., Ghena, N., Schmaedick, M. and Cheng, A., 2018. Intermittent metabolic switching, neuroplasticity and brain health. *Nature Reviews Neuroscience*, 19(2), pp.81-94.

Chapter 2- The Stages of Fasting

"I delivered a lecture on this topic- Kenny, R., 2022. *Age Proof: The New Science of Living a Longer and Healthier Life.* [S.l.]: BLINK PUBLISHING, p.163.

BDNF has been called 'a miracle grow for the human brain'- Hagerman, E. and Ratey, J., 2014. *Spark: The Revolutionary New Science of Exercise and the Brain.* New York: Little, Brown and Co.

…found to induce weight loss in lab rats by suppressing appetite- Pelleymounter, M., Cullen, M. and Wellman, C., 1995. Characteristics of BDNF-induced weight loss. *Experimental Neurology*, 131(2), pp.229-238.

…trying to refeed too quickly, leading to heart failure- Kosokov, A. and Osinin, S., 1984. *Therapeutic Fasting in Bronchial and Asthma Patients.* Siberika Publishing

When you break a long fast, do so gradually- Chavda, M., 2007. *The Hidden Power of Prayer and Fasting.* Racine: Treasures Media Inc., p.130.

…in terms of ideals, behaviour and adaptivity- Ho, K., *et al,* 1988. Fasting enhances growth hormone secretion and amplifies the complex rhythms of growth hormone secretion in man. *Journal of Clinical Investigation,* 81(4), pp.968-975.

…ghrelin could raise their levels of voluntary exercise- Mifune, H., *et al,* 2020. Voluntary exercise is motivated by ghrelin, possibly related to the central reward circuit. *Journal of Endocrinology,* 244(1), pp.123-132.

Chapter 3- Different Ways to Fast

Combining exercise and fasting in this way improves body composition- delli Paoli, G., *et al.,*

2020. Short-Term, Combined Fasting and Exercise Improves Body Composition in Healthy Males. *International Journal of Sport Nutrition and Exercise Metabolism*, 30(6), pp.386-395.

…salt can still be used to help suppress appetite- Shields, D., 2022. *A Comprehensive Guide To Fasting : Timeline, Stages & Benefits*. [online] Dr. Alexis Shields. Available at: <https://dralexisshields.com/guide-to-fasting>

…our normal healthy cellular responses in other situations."- Bennion, D., 2015. *Feast then famine – how fasting might make our cells more resilient to stress*. [online] The Conversation. Available at: <https://theconversation.com/feast-then-famine-how-fasting-might-make-our-cells-more-resilient-to-stress-38808>

…absorbed in their entire lifetime- Heim, S. and Keil, A., 2022. *Too Much Information, Too Little Time: How the Brain Separates Important from Unimportant Things in Our Fast-Paced Media World*. [online] Frontiers for Young Minds. Available at:

<https://kids.frontiersin.org/articles/10.3389/frym.2017.00023>

…equivalent to reading 175 newspapers cover to cover- Hilbert, M., 2012. How much information is there in the "information society"?. *Significance*, 9(4), pp.8-12.

…aware of good health and... living in comfort."- Wikipitaka - The Completing Tipitaka. 2022. *Kitagiri Sutta*. [online] Available at: <https://tipitaka.fandom.com/wiki/Kitagiri_Sutta>

…tells in his autobiography of a fearful time- Black Elk, Neihardt, J., Deloria, P. and DeMallie, R., 1932. *Black Elk Speaks: Being the Life Story of a Holy Man of the Oglala Sioux*. University of Nebraska Press.

…a forty day fast, undertaken for religious reasons- Kirby, T., 2006. Family mourns devout Christian who died after fasting for 23 days. *The Independent*, [online] Available at: <https://www.independent.co.uk/news/uk/this-britain/family-mourns-devout-christian-who-died-after-fasting-for-23-days-6101383.html>

…driving is not advisable for this reason- Voigt, K., et al, 2021. The Hunger Games: Homeostatic State-Dependent Fluctuations in Disinhibition Measured with a Novel Gamified Test Battery. *Nutrients*, 13(6), p.2001.

"grin and bear it."- Bragg, P. and Bragg, P., 2011. *The miracle of fasting*.

…credits intermittent fasting with reversing type two diabetes- J;, A.M.B. (2021) *Intermittent fasting: Is there a role in the treatment of diabetes? A review of the literature and guide for Primary Care Physicians, Clinical diabetes and endocrinology*. U.S. National Library of Medicine. Available at: https://pubmed.ncbi.nlm.nih.gov/33531076/

…doing nothing is the same as doing something wrong- Pirsig, R., 1991. *Lila- an inquiry into morals*. New York, NY: Bantam Books, p.436.

...to rest and realign his forces to suit the new requirements- Liedloff, J., 2004. *The Continuum Concept*. London: Penguin, p.58.

...this is having a detrimental effect on us- Hari, J., 2021. *Stolen Focus*. P.32.

I think IF has amazing potential as a therapy- Harvard Health. 2022. *Intermittent fasting: Surprising update - Harvard Health.* [online] Available at: <https://www.health.harvard.edu/blog/intermittent-fasting-surprising-update-2018062914156>

...their own body can fix it by itself."- Isabel A. Moser. How and When to Be Your Own Doctor (Best Motivational Books for Personal Development (Design Your Life)) (p. 46). Prabhat Prakashan.

Chapter 5- Fasting Difficulties and Myths

Jeanette Winterson quote- "Why I fasted for 11 days," The Guardian [online], 11.07.15

...why fasting is not very popular."- Bragg, P. and Bragg, P., 2011. *The miracle of fasting*. Santa Barbara, Calif.: Health Science.

…**what makes us happy is doing the thing that's a little bit difficult."-** Hari, J., 2021. *Stolen Focus*. P.31.

…**to invoke pain in subjects without causing lasting damage-** Benedetti, F., Thoen, W., Blanchard, C., Vighetti, S. and Arduino, C., 2013. Pain as a reward: Changing the meaning of pain from negative to positive co-activates opioid and cannabinoid systems. *Pain*, 154(3), pp.361-367.

Upton Sinclair quote- Shelton, H., 2019. *The science and fine arts of fasting*. Mockingbird Press.

…**it soon becomes the more appealing way to live."-** Burkeman, O., 2022. *Oliver Burkeman's last column: the eight secrets to a (fairly) fulfilled life.* [online] the Guardian. Available at: <https://www.theguardian.com/lifeandstyle/2020/sep/04/oliver-burkemans-last-column-the-eight-secrets-to-a-fairly-fulfilled-life>

Alan Goldhamer quote- Goldhamer, A., 2022. *Alan Goldhamer, dc: Water Fasting—The Clinical Effectiveness of Rebooting Your Body.* [online]

PubMed Central (PMC). Available at: <https://www.ncbi.nlm.nih.gov/pmc/articles/PMC4684131/>

…was found to reverse symptoms of depression- Lee, E., Park, J., Kwon, H. and Han, P., 2021. Repeated exposure with short-term behavioural stress resolves pre-existing stress-induced depressive-like behavior in mice. *Nature Communications*, 12(1).

…on a fast is controversial," says Isabel A. Moser- Moser, D. and Solomon, S., 1997. *How and When to Be Your Own Doctor?*. La Vergne: E-Kitap Projesi & Cheapest Books. P. 63

***…a cheese sandwich, which I promptly threw up**- Jones, A., 2022. Ditching the diet – how I learned to accept the body I have.* [online] the Guardian. Available at: <https://www.theguardian.com/lifeandstyle/2022/jan/01/ditching-the-diet-how-i-learned-to-accept-the-body-i-have>

Alan Goldhamer quote- Gustafson, C., 2014. *Alan Goldhamer, dc: Water Fasting—The*

Clinical Effectiveness of Rebooting Your Body.
[online] PubMed Central (PMC). Available at:
<https://www.ncbi.nlm.nih.gov/pmc/articles/PMC
4684131/>

Acknowledgements

The title *The Importance of Being Idle* is
borrowed from the song of the same name by Noel
Gallagher, who probably borrowed it from Oscar
Wilde.

Mailing list for new books-
https://mailchi.mp/c4f6565242a6/alexandervladim

www.ingramcontent.com/pod-product-compliance
Lightning Source LLC
Chambersburg PA
CBHW071011250726

48653CB00005B/1582